NATURAL BEAUTY

Here is a programme for regaining and
preserving the glowing good looks that
Nature intended you to have.

By the same author
THE VITAMIN FACT FINDER
THE NATURAL FOODS HEALTHY BABY COOKBOOK
THE 'HERE'S HEALTH' COOKBOOK

NATURAL BEAUTY

The Healthy Way to
Radiant Good Looks

Carol Hunter

THORSONS PUBLISHING GROUP
Wellingborough, Northamptonshire

First Edition 1979
Second Edition, completely revised
and updated 1988

British Library Cataloguing in Publication Data

Hunter, Carol
Natural beauty: the healthy way to radiant
good looks.—2nd ed.
1. Beauty, Personal   2. Diet   3. Food, Natural
I. Title
646.7'2   RA778

ISBN 0-7225-0934-0

Printed and Bound in Great Britain

3 5 7 9 10 8 6 4 2

CONTENTS

CHAPTER ONE

WHAT IS NATURAL BEAUTY?

You could spend hundreds of pounds on trying to improve your looks with expensive cosmetics and beauty salon treatments, only to find, at the end of it all, that you looked little better than before you started. You might pass as a beauty from a distance, but anyone taking a closer look would be in for a shock. This is because the best such measures can achieve is to mask any imperfections or blemishes you may have – they can never give you those basic attributes which go to make up a natural beauty.

Natural beauty is a rare quality which has as much to do with clear skin, bright eyes and shining hair as it does with perfect features. And while you cannot change your features, you can work towards attaining these other basic requirements of natural beauty.

The trouble is that although most people are concerned about their looks, few are prepared to put in any effort when it comes to improving their appearance. Yet, as you will find when you read this book, many of the measures advocated for beauty will also benefit your health. And a basic beauty routine, once you get into the swing of it, will take up only a few minutes of your time each day.

The earlier you start to care for your looks the better, and if mothers were more fastidious about introducing their children to a beauty care routine, they might encounter fewer beauty problems during the teens. Don't give up hope, however, if this period of your life is little more than a hazy memory, for it is never too late to start beauty treatment. The results may be less spectacular, but you'll find that perseverance will pay off whatever your age.

GIVING NATURE A HELPING HAND

Some people feel that nature should be left to her own devices when it comes to their appearance, but there are ways in which you can improve your looks without compromising a belief in doing things the natural way. And, as you will see later, beauty is closely related to your health and diet, as well as to how much sleep, fresh air and exercise you get.

Certainly there is an element of vanity involved in caring for your looks, but an attractive appearance not only pleases the beholder. It also gives the person concerned an added feeling of confidence which is reflected in other areas of her life. You know yourself how much better you feel mentally when you know that you are looking your best.

Cosmetics can play their part in natural living too. The cosmetic business is a large and lucrative one, and the companies in this field make millions of pounds from pandering to the vanity of both men and women. Every year more weird and wonderful products emerge from the laboratory, packed full of chemicals, decked out in elaborate packaging, and complete with nebulous promises of eternal youth and longer-lasting beauty. It is ironic that many people carefully avoid refined processed foods in their diet, while blithely applying synthetic cosmetics to their body.

There are trends in beauty, as in most things, and recent years have seen a tremendous upsurge in the popularity of natural cosmetics. These are made from herbs, plants and other natural ingredients, many of which have been used for hundreds of years for their beautifying properties. The manufacturers of these products try, as far as possible, to avoid the use of synthetic ingredients and chemical additives, believing that natural ingredients work in harmony with the body. It is an idea with undoubted aesthetic appeal, and one to which the cosmetic market has been quick to latch on. Many of the large companies produce so-called natural cosmetics, which only too often are synthetic products with herbal ingredients added. However, until the contents of cosmetics have to be declared (as they already are in America), there is no way of knowing just what has gone into a particular product.

LOOK IN YOUR HEALTH FOOD SHOP

The best hunting ground for natural cosmetics is your health food shop. Here you will find a wide range of products, many of which have an interesting and appealing story behind them. Some may have been produced by hand in the maker's own kitchen, while others will have been made from herbs and plants freshly picked on the very day of manufacture. Such products are likely to be as near to natural as possible, although it is impractical to expect a product to be completely natural since not only would it go mouldy, but its performance and consistency would probably be unacceptable. It is extremely difficult to preserve a product without resorting to chemicals, although such ingredients as essential oils help act as natural preservatives. Most manufacturers are obliged to make use of very small amounts of synthetic preservatives. As one natural cosmetic manufacturer put it 'our products are 99.9 per cent natural.'

Among the natural ingredients, you'll find such appetizing substances as cucumber, honey, fruit juices and vegetable oils. Herbs like rosemary, chamomile and lavender are popular ingredients, while essential oils (obtained by distilling flowers) are used to impart a delicate fragrance and to enliven the circulation.

The small companies in this market believe in letting their products speak for themselves. Most don't spend thousands of pounds on fancy packaging or extensive advertising (they couldn't afford to!), which means they can sell their cosmetics at prices which compare very favourably with those on the mass market. The last few years have seen an influx of natural cosmetics from America, but when considering such products it is worth bearing in mind that the American health food trade is far less scrupulous than the British about accepting conventional cosmetics with additional natural extracts. This means, for instance, that when an American product claims to be natural, it may contain a larger proportion of preservatives, as well as mineral oils and synthetic detergents. American cosmetics have by law to carry an ingredients list, although there is still no way of knowing sometimes whether a particular ingredient (e.g. vitamin E) is derived from natural or synthetic sources. Ingredients which have numbers signify laboratory origins, but some of the long names (e.g. hexadecanol) are natural in origin.

British cosmetics are much more likely to use vegetable rather than mineral oils (the latter, a by-product of the petroleum industry, is considerably cheaper but is less easily absorbed by the skin); beeswax instead of cheaper waxes; and naturally derived perfumes. Another major difference is in the use of animal extracts, with American cosmetics being more likely to use these, such as elastin and collagen (see page 135).

The subject of animal testing is an emotive one, but it is a fact that almost all cosmetic ingredients – even if not the final product – will have been tested on animals at some stage. Manufacturers are required by law to show that their cosmetics will not cause harm to humans under normal conditions of use, although there is no specific requirement to test on animals. Most manufacturers will in fact protect themselves by using standard animal tests, although the number has fallen from 31.3 thousand in 1980 to 17.5 thousand in 1984 (this accounts for 0.56 per cent of animal experiments).

One of the most common tests for general toxicity is LD50, (lethal dose 50 per cent), in which animals are force-fed the test substance to establish the dose which will kill 50 per cent of them. Anything from 30 to 100 animals may be needed to test one substance. The Draize test is another common one, and in this case the test substance is dropped into the unprotected eyes of the animals (usually rabbits) to assess the effect over a period of several days. The Draize test is also used on the skin, when a patch of skin is shaved and the test substance applied and covered, then left for between 24 and 72 hours to assess any skin damage. Humane researchers are looking for alternatives to Draize, and a three year grant, funded by the Dr. Hadwen Research Trust, has now been extended for a further year to allow research to continue. Two techniques, neither of which uses live animals, are being investigated, one using tissue from dead rabbits, and the other using corneas obtained from the slaughterhouse.

Cosmetic manufacturers may be able to claim that their products have not been tested on animals (as do those under the 'cruelty free' banner), but it is a different matter when it comes to raw ingredients. Most companies if questioned will admit the likelihood of ingredients having been tested on animals at some stage, even if it was many years ago. And while one supplier may not test a particular material, another may be testing an identical one (for instance, jojoba was subjected to the LD50 test in America in 1979). Even widely used natural ingredients like lanolin and beeswax will have been tested at some stage.

In America, where there are stringent laws relating to product liability, manufacturers tend to test products on both animals and humans. And French law apparently forbids the use of human volunteers, so manufacturers will use animals. The EEC Cosmetics Directive of 1976 requires animal studies on ingredients, although discussions since then mean that safety-in-use data may now be acceptable for some ingredients. The Animals (Scientific Procedures) Act passed in 1986 does not deal specifically with cosmetics, and certainly does not ban animal experiments, but it does mean that applications for a licence for cosmetic testing must be approved by the Animal Procedures Committee. It is as yet too early to tell whether this will mean a reduction in animal testing.

In the meantime the only legal restraint on animal testing is the Cruelty to Animals Act of 1876. This merely states that all laboratories in which pain is likely to be inflicted on animals must be licensed, and that all experiments must be 'for the stated purpose of acquisition of knowledge that would be helpful to human beings.' Not only is the law itself far too lax, but only a handful of Home Office inspectors is employed to oversee more than 600 laboratories.

While manufacturers are clearly in a very difficult position when it comes to avoiding animal testing, many in the health food market do at least avoid ingredients derived from animals in their cosmetics.

NOT FORGETTING THE MEN
No beauty book would be complete without at least a mention of men and their looks. Gone are the days when men were considered effeminate if they so much as used a deodorant, and the proliferation of aftershaves, hair lotions, skin care products and even make-up, designed with men in mind, suggests that the male population is at last admitting an interest in its appearance.

Most of the problems men encounter with their skin, for instance dry skin, cuts and rashes, are undoubtedly due to the daily ritual of shaving. Because men (or most men at any rate!) do not wear make up, a special cleanser is less important, and a good pure soap can be used instead. A moisturizer, preferably one free from perfume, helps cope with cracked, rough or red skin.

Shaving foams consist primarily of detergent, with lubricants and emollients (usually stearic acid) added, while shaving creams have an added pearlizing agent, plus ingredients to thicken and perfume the cream. Such products can be very harsh and drying, although there are now one or two gentler and more natural shaving products on the market.

Aftershave lotions are one of the best sellers among men's toiletries (although usually bought by women rather than men!). These also tend to be over-astringent and drying because they contain a large proportion of alcohol, with added perfume and oil derivatives. For skins that react adversely, experiment with a natural aftershave, or try spraying with evian water in an atomizer.

Other common problems such as dandruff, broken nails or greasy hair could all be eliminated if men took a little care of themselves. So, for those men who want to look good – the advice contained in this book is just as relevant to you as it is to women, and while no one expects you to 'go the whole hog', you could at least carry out the basic rudiments without compromising your dignity.

CHAPTER TWO

BEAUTY IS MORE THAN SKIN DEEP

To the trained eye, your skin, hair, eyes, nails and teeth all have a story to tell. The condition they are in gives a good indication both of your general state of health, and of any deficiencies in your diet. For instance, when somebody is under the weather their hair, skin and eyes quickly lose their natural lustre, and instead look dull and tired. In the same way, such common beauty problems as broken nails or falling hair can all too often be traced back to an imbalance in the diet (in these two cases, a deficiency of the B vitamins).

Just as diet and health are closely related, so too are diet and beauty. And, as we have just seen, health also has a close bearing on beauty. What you eat (or don't eat) has a dramatic effect on your outward appearance as well as on your physical well-being.

EATING FOR BEAUTY

What is the right sort of diet to choose for improved looks? Ideally it is one which supplies a sufficient quantity of all the nutrients essential to both health and beauty. At the end of this chapter you will find a chart listing the nutrients of particular importance to beauty, together with their main sources. As you will see from this list, when this is translated in terms of food it represents a diet based on wholefoods and incorporates plenty of fresh raw fruit and vegetables.

Wholefoods are those which are as near as possible to their natural state, and as such they contain the maximum amount of nutrients. These foods have not been subjected to rigorous refining processes which destroy many valuable nutrients, and where possible wholefoods are free from the artificial additives which are so widely used in refined foods. It is by choosing wholefoods, and avoiding the many processed foods on the market, that you can build up health and vitality through diet.

A wholefood diet would include the following:

WHOLEMEAL FLOUR

This contains 100 per cent of the original wheat grain, complete with vitamins E, B, A, protein, unsaturated fat and natural roughage. During the production of white flour many valuable nutrients are lost (including the wheat germ and bran, which are removed). Since only four of these nutrients are replaced by synthetic equivalents, the natural balance of the wheat grain is completely upset. Wholemeal flour is also free from additives of any description, unlike white flour which contains a long list of chemicals designed to improve its appearance, texture and keeping properties. Even wholemeal bread is allowed to contain a certain number of additives like emulsifiers, stabilizers and preservatives, so the answer is really to bake your own. You will find that with a little practice wholemeal flour can be used for all your baking requirements, and once you've adjusted to the new taste you'll enjoy the improved flavour.

WHOLEGRAIN CEREALS

Just as wholemeal flour contains more goodness than white, so the wholegrain cereals are richer in nutrients than their refined equivalents. Wholegrains are rich in vitamins E and B (especially riboflavin, thiamine, niacin, pantothenic acid and B6), as well as being a good source of protein and natural roughage. Into this category come breakfast cereals, pasta, rice, and less well-known grains like rye, barley and buckwheat.

RAW SUGAR

No sugar is good for you, and since a high sugar intake is linked with such diseases as diabetes and coronary thrombosis, you should cut down on sugar in any form. While white sugar provides nothing but calories, raw sugar does contain small quantities of vitamins and minerals, in particular calcium, iron, phosphorus and the B vitamins. Since raw sugar is stronger in taste than white, you'll also find that you need to use less of it to achieve the same degree of sweetness. Other natural sweeteners to use in place of sugar are honey, molasses and dried fruit, all of which provide valuable nutrients.

VEGETABLE FATS

A high intake of saturated fats, chiefly from animal sources, has been strongly linked with coronary and vascular diseases. The Royal College of Physicians has recommended people to cut their total fat intake by one third, and to switch to those fats which are unsaturated, i.e. vegetable fats. Coconut oil is one vegetable fat which is highly saturated (although it is widely used by food manufacturers), so when buying vegetable oil or margarine it is worth checking that it is in fact unsaturated. The oils highest in polyunsaturates are, in descending order, safflower, sunflower, corn, cotton seed, soya, wheat germ, sesame and peanut.

Anyone who is inclined to greasy skin or hair should take care to limit their fat intake, although fats should never be totally excluded from the diet since they are required to maintain healthy cells and skin structure. Conversely, those with dry skin or hair should add a tablespoonful of vegetable oil to their daily diet, preferably in the form of salad dressing, since fried foods simply add unwanted calories and make foods less digestible.

FRUIT AND VEGETABLES

These are an excellent source of a wide range of vitamins,

minerals and roughage, especially when eaten raw, since cooking destroys many nutrients. Eat as many of these foods as you can, making sure that you include at least one salad each day.

PROCEED WITH CAUTION

Having chosen the ingredients of your diet with care, you must then proceed to prepare and cook them carefully if you are to avoid unnecessary destruction of nutrients. Vitamins and minerals are extremely unstable substances, and can easily be destroyed by such common factors as storage, exposure to air, heat or water.

Foods should be cooked as and when they are required, rather than being left to soak or to stand around. It is healthier to roast or grill foods than to fry them, and to cook at low temperatures for the shortest possible time. Always serve at once, rather than keeping hot or reheating.

Particular care should be taken with vegetables, which should not be peeled before cooking since many nutrients are contained in and immediately under the skin. Wash and chop vegetables immediately prior to cooking, and use the minimum amount of liquid: vegetables do not need to be immersed – ½ pt. (275ml) of liquid is ample to cook vegetables for four people. Plunge vegetables straight into boiling water, and cook for the minimum length of time. When cooked, vegetables should retain some of their original crunchiness. Reserve the cooking liquid, which is by now rich in nutrients, for use in soups, casseroles or drinks.

PLANNING A MENU

A basic menu would be as follows:

Breakfast:
  Freshly squeezed fruit juice
  Muesli served with wheat germ, fresh fruit and
  unsweetened yogurt

Wholemeal bread and honey
Milk or herbal tea

Lunch:
  Mixed vegetable salad with a dressing of yogurt and
    lemon juice, or cider vinegar and vegetable oil
  Wholemeal bread and low fat cheese or lean meat
  Fresh fruit
  Fruit juice or herb tea

Supper:
  Home-made soup
  Egg or cheese dish, or meat or fish, served with lightly
    cooked vegetables
  Fresh fruit salad or a fruit-based dessert
  Decaffeinated coffee or herb tea

In addition to this you should drink plenty of liquids, in
the form of five or six glasses of water or fruit juice daily.

VITAMINS FOR BEAUTY
As you will see from the chart, the vitamins each have a part
to play in the way you look.
  Vitamin A is essential for healthy eyesight, especially at
night time. Those who use their eyes a lot, such as typists or
draughtsmen, need extra quantities of this vitamin. Problems with the eyes are often a sign of a vitamin A
deficiency. A shortage of this vitamin can also cause the
skin to become clogged, leading to blemishes and rough
skin resembling gooseflesh, the latter being most common
on the upper arms, the knees and thighs.
  The Vitamin B Complex is involved in controlling skin
secretions, and as such is vital for healthy skin and hair. The
B vitamins also help counteract stress, which takes a heavy
toll on our appearance. The best source of the complex is

brewer's yeast, which not only contains the whole B complex, but has 14 minerals, 17 amino acids, and a high proportion of the protein needed for healthy hair and skin. Take it in tablet form, or add the powder to cereals, stews, baked dishes, etc.

Vitamin C helps to purify and revitalize the blood stream and so is essential for good skin. Since this vitamin cannot be stored in the body, it is vital to obtain a daily intake.

Vitamin D's prime role is the part it plays in bone formation, together with the minerals calcium and phosphorus. It is also needed for healthy teeth, and a deficiency appears to be linked with dental decay.

Vitamin E is one of the latest discoveries in the beauty field, and has had many miraculous claims made for it. An increasing number of women swear by its ability to heal scar tissue, and to delay and diminish wrinkles. Vitamin E is applied externally for cosmetic purposes, but should also be eaten for a better complexion resulting from improved circulation. Wheat germ is one of the best sources, and is also rich in protein and vitamin A.

OTHER IMPORTANT FACTORS
Diet is not the only factor with a direct effect on your looks. Almost as important is the need for adequate sleep, fresh air and exercise, all of these being vital for looks as well as for health. Proper elimination and correct posture also have an important part to play in the way you look.

SLEEP
Although individual requirements vary considerably, most people find that around eight hours' sleep a night is the ideal amount. If you have difficulty in sleeping, try taking a warm drink, such as hot milk with honey or molasses, before going to bed. Avoid burning the candle at both ends, since this will not only make you feel tense and

irritable, but will be reflected in dark bags and lines around the eyes.

FRESH AIR
Breathing is something we do automatically and unconsciously, but in fact it's a pity that people don't think more about their breathing. If they did they would find that their usual rate of breathing is shallow and does not make full use of the lungs. Breathing should be deep, relaxed and regular – correct breathing stimulates the circulation by increasing the flow of oxygen around the body. Make sure your rooms are well-ventilated (including the bedroom), and try to get some fresh air every day. If you have central heating, use a humidifier or place a bowl of water near the heater to maintain the correct humidity.

ELIMINATION
Constipation gives skin a grey, tired look, dulls the eyes, and makes the hair lank and lifeless. If you are eating a wholefood diet you should have little trouble with constipation. However, if you do suffer at all, include two tablespoonsful of natural bran in your daily diet, by adding it to cereals, soups, stews, drinks, or using it in baking.

EXERCISE
Exercise and keeping fit have become something of an obsession in the '80s, and perhaps this is a reaction to the sedentary lifestyle so many of us lead. Opportunities for exercise have never been better, with ample facilities available for all kinds of sport, yoga, dancing, swimming, weight training and so on.

When you look at the advantages to be gained from regular exercise it is a wonder that everybody is not super fit but, as with losing weight or giving up cigarettes, it is a question of first finding the initial motivation and self discipline. Some people start off with good intentions but

are then discouraged because they do not see any im-
mediate results, but if you can get over the initial aches and
stiffness and begin to feel the benefit of exercise, it
suddenly becomes a pleasure rather than a pain.

Regular exercise has the following benefits:
- it generates more energy and lessens fatigue. Experts say
  that an unfit body is only 27 per cent efficient in its use of
  available energy.
- it increases general alertness and makes one better able
  to cope with stress.
- it affects the blood fats and lipoproteins which decrease
  the overall risk of heart and arterial disease.
- it increases the body's basal metabolic rate (by as much
  as 25 per cent for 12 hours or more, and by ten per cent
  for the next two days). This is of particular interest to
  those who find it hard to lose weight, since a higher
  metabolic rate means the body burns up calories faster.
- it improves body shape. Exercise increases the amount
  of glycogen in the muscles (the form sugar is stored in)
  and accustoms the body to using more oxygen, so fat
  tissue is replaced by lean.
- it increases suppleness, strength and stamina, depending on what sort of exercise you choose (see below).
- it improves blood circulation.
- it tones up many other body systems.

Before you start an exercise programme you need to give
some thought to what sort of sport or activity you would
most enjoy (you are more likely to keep at it if it is
something you like doing). If you have any doubts about
your health, or if you are over 30 and generally unfit, it is
important to have a medical check up first. For maximum
benefit it is a good idea to choose more than one form of
exercise, so that you combine those which improve
strength, suppleness and stamina. For instance, jogging is
good for building up stamina but does not improve

suppleness. Both yoga and dance, on the other hand, are excellent for improving suppleness, and this is worth building up and maintaining as it decreases dramatically with age.

The latest exercise craze is aerobics, which aims to get more oxygen through the system. It strengthens the heart, lungs, blood vessels and other organs through sustained use of oxygen. Aerobic exercise is exercise which is maintained at a steady, vigorous level for a considerable period of time, i.e. for at least five minutes, but preferably 10 or more. Short, sharp exercise like sprinting simply uses up oxygen stored in the muscles, while over-strenuous exercise (indicated by extreme breathlessness) means that the body cannot supply the volume of oxygen required.

Good examples of aerobic exercise are jogging, brisk walking, swimming (an excellent, all round exercise), hiking, aerobic classes, mountaineering, volleyball, digging the garden, and cross country ski-ing (not available to many of us, but the best of all aerobic exercises).

Weight training is another form of exercise which is popular at the moment. This does not, as the name might imply, result in overdeveloped muscles, but it does firm and strengthen them thereby protecting the joints and improving general body shape, especially those areas most resistant to weight loss, such as the thighs, buttocks and upper arms. Most gymnasiums will show you what to do and will work out an individual programme of exercises with you, and they should check your pulse rate (and possibly your blood pressure) before and after a session. Weight training should not be confused with weight lifting: in the former, exercises are performed with the added resistance of small weights, either strapped to the wrist or ankle, or used as dumbells or barbells. Weight training also makes use of fixed weight stations or multi-gym equipment, which tones the muscles by offering various forms of resistance when a particular movement (e.g. pushing) is made. Ideally weight training should be undertaken in conjunction with aerobic exercise.

Whatever form of exercise you decide to try, you need to start very gradually, always listening to your body and pushing it when you can, but stopping at once if you suffer any pain or other warning signs. Always warm up first with a few stretching exercises, and always wear loose, comfortable clothing and the correct footwear. As you become fitter, so you can build up gradually. For instance, if you are jogging, you start off by alternating running and walking, and then gradually lengthen the periods of running and decrease the periods of walking. One guide is that you should be able to hold a conversation while exercising – even if a bit breathlessly!

A safety measure which is especially recommended for women over 35 and men over 45, particularly those who drink or smoke heavily or are more than 14lbs overweight, is to take note of your pulse rate. This is a simplified version of a scientific method devised by the Cardiac Research Unit at London's City Gym. What you do is take the figure 200, subtract from it your age, and add a handicap of 40 if you are unfit. As soon as you begin to tire or to feel breathless while exercising, stop and take your pulse for one minute. If it is racing above your safety limit, you should stop at once, and proceed more cautiously. As you become more fit you can gradually reduce your handicap of 40 until you are left without one at all. However, if you are over 45 years old, it is advisable to retain a handicap of 20. If you suffer from high blood pressure and are taking drugs to beat the condition, do not use this method as a gauge, since the drugs may disguise a true pulse reading.

Exercising for between 15 and 30 minutes three times a week is enough to keep you fit. However, one or two sessions are said to have little effect, while four sessions are said to be three times more effective than three sessions.

The following exercises can be used as a gentle introduction to a get-fit routine, or as a supplement, but they are not intended as a substitute.

Begin first thing in the morning, before you even get out of bed, by really stretching your body from head to toe. Then relax for a few minutes (without going back to sleep!). Repeat this exercise when you get up.

With the following exercises start off with a few minutes each day, gradually building up the length of time.

Arms
Stand upright, feet together, and swing your arms backwards and forwards as high and as hard as possible.

Bust
With your arms level with your shoulders, elbows out, press the palms of your hands together. Count to ten and then relax.

Stomach
This is one of the worst areas as far as sagging muscles go. Lie on your back on the floor, hands by your side and legs out straight. Lift your legs slowly until they are at right angles to the ground. Lower them slowly; when your feet are six inches from the floor, hold this position for a count of six before continuing to lower them to the ground.

Waist
Stand with your feet apart, hands stretched above your head. Circle the top part of your body, trying to touch the floor and then reach up as high as you can. Don't bend your knees. Repeat, rotating the body in the other direction.

Back
Lie on your front, arms bent, and with your head resting on your hands. With your legs straight, lift one at a time as high up behind you as you can. Hold and then slowly lower to the floor. Repeat with the other leg.

Bottom
Sit on the floor, arms and legs out straight in front of you. 'Walk' backwards and forwards on your bottom.

Legs
Stand with feet together, arms by your sides. Bend your knees while keeping your heels on the floor. Repeat three times, then raise your heels off the ground and bend right down as low as you can. Rise slowly, bringing hands up over your head with arms straight.

POSTURE
Many a potential beauty has been marred by poor posture. In fact this must be the most common of all beauty problems, although it is not often recognized as such. Standing, walking and sitting incorrectly not only spoil your looks, but put an unnecessary strain on the bones and joints which can result in backache and other postural complaints. Incorrect posture can also limit the supply of oxygen if the chest and lungs are cramped, and can be involved in digestive troubles. Good posture, on the other hand, helps to improve the figure.

The first step towards good posture is to learn how to stand correctly, and to achieve this it helps to position yourself in front of a full-length mirror. Stand up straight, and imagine a thread running up through your body and head which lifts and stretches the whole body. If you find this difficult to imagine, hang a piece of weighted string from the top of your mirror as a guide. Pull your stomach in, tuck your buttocks under, with chest high, and shoulders pulled back but relaxed. If it feels uncomfortable, this is a sure sign that your usual stance leaves much to be desired.

This is the posture you should maintain for walking too. Step out with your toes straight ahead, and your arms swinging in a relaxed way as you walk. Move from the thighs rather than the hips, remembering to keep your back straight. Hold your head straight too, with chin up, and breathe deeply. When you are sitting, try and sit upright – you'll find this easier on a hardbacked chair, than on one of the inviting, soft-cushioned, modern lounging chairs. Correct posture while sitting is particularly important for those with sedentary jobs. Check that your desk and chair are the correct height – your feet should rest flat on the floor, with your bottom right to the back of the chair, and your back straight.

It is impossible to break the habits of a lifetime overnight, and the only way you are likely to improve your posture is to take regular checks on the way you stand, walk and sit. Whenever it occurs to you, check to see what your faults are, and correct them as described above. You will find that it becomes easier with practice, so it is worth persevering.

ENEMIES OF BEAUTY
Other habits that are likely to have an adverse affect on your looks as well as your health are alcohol, smoking, and stress. **Alcohol** not only uses up the B vitamins which, as already mentioned, play an important part in beauty, but it also encourages the appearance of thread veins, which are almost impossible to eradicate. **Smoking** is said to encourage the formation of wrinkles, and although there is no scientific proof of this, it is a fact that each cigarette uses up 25mg of vitamin C. Since this is almost equivalent to the minimum recommended daily intake (which is 30mg), anyone who smokes heavily is almost certain to be short of this important nutrient.

Stress, of course, is less under our control, especially in the high-pressured society in which most of us live. However, stress can be conquered to a large extent if the correct mental attitude is adopted. Many people find that the regular practice of yoga, meditation or relaxation techniques helps them to combat stress, and anybody who is subjected to undue stress in their daily life would be well advised to enquire about these. Otherwise, you will find that the signs of tension will be all too obvious, in a drawn appearance with early wrinkles – not the laughter lines which can add character to a face, but the worried frown lines which impair your looks.

FOODS FOR BEAUTY

Nutrient and Main Function	Main Dietary Sources
VITAMIN A for healthy hair and eyes, resistance to infections (which can lead to acne), suntanning. Also counteracts dandruff, dry skin and wrinkle formation. Needed for healthy circulation.	Fish liver oils, liver and other offal, dairy produce, eggs, carrots, spinach, watercress, apricots.
VITAMIN B COMPLEX for healthy hair and skin. A deficiency can lead to greasy hair, dandruff, dry skin, redness and irritations, wrinkles and poor hair growth.	Wholewheat bread and flour, wholegrains, liver, wheat germ, brown rice, molasses, meat, fish, brewer's yeast.
VITAMIN C for hair, eyes and teeth, resistance to infection, healing of wounds, firm skin tissues. Dry skin and thread veins can be caused by a deficiency.	Green vegetables, fresh fruit, especially citrus fruits, blackcurrants, rose hips, green peppers.
VITAMIN D for healthy teeth, bones and nails. Essential for the assimilation of calcium and phosphorus.	Fish liver oils, eggs, butter, margarine.
VITAMIN E to prevent wrinkles, dry skin, brown age spots and dandruff. Helps to improve circulation and healing of scars.	Wholewheat bread, wholegrains, wheat germ, eggs, nuts, vegetable oils

Nutrient and Main Function	Main Dietary Sources
PROTEIN for healthy hair, skin, teeth and nails. For firm skin tissues.	Meat, fish, dairy produce, nuts, pulses, wheat germ, brewer's yeast.
FATS to counteract dry skin and hair and for assimilation of fat soluble vitamins A, D, E, and K.	Butter, margarine, vegetable oils, nuts, egg yolk.
CALCIUM and PHOSPHORUS work together for healthy teeth, hair, nails and bones.	*Calcium:* eggs, dairy produce, green vegetables. *Phosphorus:* As calcium, plus nuts, wheat germ, meat, pulses.

CHAPTER THREE

ALL YOU NEED TO KNOW ABOUT SKIN CARE

Skin care is rather like health – it is something we tend to ignore until signs of neglect begin to show. It is only when a revealing glance in the mirror one day reveals wrinkles, spots or blemishes which never used to be there that, in a sudden panic, we resolve to pay more attention to our poor old face – by which time, of course, it takes extra care and effort to repair the damage, because with beauty (as with health) prevention is easier than cure.

Proper care of the skin is vital at any age. When you are young, it helps to prevent such common teenage problems as greasy skin and acne, while as you grow older it is important to counteract the increasing dryness of the skin. You can have a beautiful skin at any age if you know how to care for it.

When we talk about skin care we usually refer to the face because this area, more than any other, needs care and attention (we'll get round to the other areas later in the chapter). Your face is constantly exposed to the elements, even in the depths of winter when the rest of you is well-wrapped up. That is why the face is one of the first parts to show signs of ageing.

GETTING TO KNOW YOUR SKIN

Although the skin is the most obvious part of the body, surprisingly few people are aware of its structure, or of the many important functions it performs. The skin forms a protective barrier against harmful bacteria and infections. At the same time, it is a means of eliminating waste matter from the body, in the form of excess water, toxins, and carbon dioxide. The skin also has a part to play as a sense organ, in regulating the body temperature, in respiration, and in the metabolic processes of the body.

The skin is divided into three layers, and it is from the innermost layer that the various glands, including the oil and sweat glands, penetrate to the surface to eliminate waste matter. This inner layer, which is based on the fatty adipose tissue of the lower dermis, also acts as a cushion for the rest of the skin. It contains the finely distributed muscles of the skin which are involved in regulating body temperature. It is when these muscles contract that goose-flesh is formed on the surface of the skin.

The most important function of the middle skin layer, known as the dermis, is respiration. It is here that the countless tiny blood vessels, or capillaries, end in finely drawn networks, from where they feed the upper layer of skin which contains no blood vessels. It is the dermis which determines skin tone.

The third, or outer layer of the skin is the epidermis, which ranges in thickness from 1/20th of an inch on the palms and soles, to 1/200th of an inch on the face. The epidermis consists of several layers of cells, the outer layers being constantly shed as new layers grow up to replace them. It is this skin layer which contains the nerve endings, and the oil and sweat glands also open in the epidermis.

FIRST THINGS FIRST
How, then, do you begin to care for this complex organ which is your skin? Before you can take any steps to improve your complexion, you must first decide what skin type you have. Although the same basic rules apply to all types, certain modifications need to be made, as you will see from the chart at the end of this chapter.

The simple way to identify your skin type if you do not instantly recognize it from the descriptions in the chart, is to position yourself in daylight with a mirror (a magnifying one if you feel brave enough). Wash your face with warm water and a little mild soap, then pat dry. Take a tissue and press it to your face, concentrating on the area around the nose and the chin. If your skin is greasy there will be definite traces of oil on the tissue. A dry skin, on the other hand, will feel taut and stretched, while a normal skin will show little or no reaction. A combination skin is one which combines the characteristics of a greasy skin with those of a dry or normal one. Usually the centre panel of the face (i.e. the forehead, nose and chin) is inclined to be greasy since this area contains more sebaceous glands than any other area of the body. At the same time, the skin on the cheeks is dry. This is the type of skin most commonly found in Britain. If there is little difference between the two areas, you can treat your skin as normal. However, if the difference is marked you need to treat each area separately, as indicated on the chart on page 60. Your skin type can in fact change from time to time (due to such influences as age, weather and atmosphere) so it is worth monitoring it fairly regularly.

Even though it is possible to divide skin into one of these four categories, you will find that your skin may react very differently to that of somebody else with apparently the same skin type. For this reason the choice of cosmetics is a very individual matter, and the only way to find a product that suits you is to try many different types. Use any new cosmetic for at least two weeks to allow your skin time to adjust to it. If you then find the product unsuitable, progress to another one, always choosing cosmetics designed specifically for your skin type.

Whichever one of the four categories mentioned above you come into, you may also suffer from sensitive skin, in which case you are probably well aware of it already! This is the skin which over-reacts, for instance coming out in blotches and redness the moment you get overanxious or overexcited. The best treatment for such a skin is preventive. This means avoiding detergents, harsh products, and those which are highly coloured or perfumed. Always do a patch test on the inside of the elbow or behind the ear for a few days before using any new product on the face or scalp. It is also particularly important to avoid water which is too hot or too cold, and to protect the face from extreme weather conditions. For further advice on sensitivity to cosmetics, see page 55.

ESTABLISHING A ROUTINE

If you really want to improve your complexion you must establish a daily routine over an indefinite period – unfortunately a beautiful skin does not materialize overnight! Talk of routine may sound tedious, especially if you've been getting away with soap and water for years without any untoward effect, but it is really a small price to pay for longer-lasting beauty.

There are three basic steps in a skin care programme, which should be repeated night and morning. Once you get into the habit, you will find that they take no more than a few minutes of your time.

CLEANSING AND TONING

First and foremost, you must keep your skin thoroughly cleansed, for it is inadequate cleansing which is responsible for many skin problems. Don't be deceived if your skin *looks* clean – you'll be amazed at how much hidden dirt appears on the cotton wool when you use a good cleanser. Proper cleansing not only removes all the dust, dirt and make up which accumulate during the day, it also stops the oil-secreting sebaceous glands from getting clogged up, which can lead to spots and blackheads. This means that cleansing is especially important for greasy skins, to remove pore-clogging oil and dead cells.

There seem to be two distinct camps when it comes to cleansing, namely those who swear by soap and water, and those who would not dream of using it. Many women do find that soap makes their skin feel sensitive and taut, and this is because soap is highly alkaline, and temporarily alters the skin chemistry (the skin has a natural acid mantle, with a pH factor of about 6.5).

The usual ingredients of soap are vegetable or animal fats (e.g. rendered beef fat), and an alkali such as potassium or caustic soda. Commercial soaps are all similar, although the more expensive, smoother textured soaps will have undergone extra milling processes. Health food shops sell some soaps based on vegetable oils, chiefly palm kernel and coconut oils, and these may also include more natural extracts, such as oils of lavender or rosemary.

Soapless cleansing bars are kinder to the skin than soap, because the alkaline and detergent ingredients have been replaced with alternatives that maintain the Ph balance of the skin. Like soap, these products are designed to produce a lather in water.

A wide variety of cleansing products is available, and the sort you choose should be governed by your skin type. A dry skin, for instance, will benefit from a creamy cleansing lotion which has a larger proportion of oil to water, whereas a greasier skin is better with a light cleansing milk, which has a higher proportion of water than oil ingredients to give it a liquid consistency.

You should give your skin a thorough cleansing every evening, and then remove all vestiges of the cleanser with cotton wool soaked in warm water or toner (see below). Your skin does not need to be deep cleansed again in the morning, and a good wipe over with cotton wool soaked in toner will be sufficient to remove surface grease. When applying a cleanser or any other lotion to the face and neck, always use an upward and outward motion. This prevents the skin from being stretched in the wrong direction, and also stimulates the circulation of blood which nourishes the skin. The only exception to this rule is a toner, which should be gently patted on to the skin. Extra care should be taken when cleansing around the nostrils, since this is the oiliest part of the face. Include the eye area, but treat it with care since the skin here is very thin and delicate.

Having thoroughly cleansed your skin, now is the time to apply a toner or astringent. Since astringents have a higher alcohol content than toners (alcohol having a drying effect), these are more suited to greasy skins. However, even a greasy skin needs only a mild astringent, or flakiness may result. Both a toner and an astringent serve the same purpose, namely to remove the last traces of cleanser, to freshen the skin and close the pores.

Those who say their skin does not feel really clean unless they wash with water should try using a toner, which has a more invigorating effect. If you are still not convinced, settle for one of the deep-acting, liquid cleansers which are washed rather than wiped off. If you're using water, it should always be tepid, since extremes of temperature could encourage the formation of thread veins. When you have washed and patted dry your face, apply a toner as described above.

MOISTURIZERS
Last but not least comes the moisturizer, and it is this which helps the skin retain its youthful look, by forming a film to offset unwanted evaporation of water. A moisturizer gives moisture to the skin cells, thus lubricating and softening them. Whether your skin is dry or greasy, it still needs regular moisturizing, and this is a habit to acquire early in life, since the skin begins to lose its natural moisture and elasticity as early as twenty years old. During the day a moisturizer applied under make up helps to protect the skin against the elements, while at the same time holding in the skin's natural moisture.

When caring for your face it is easy to forget your neck, especially during the winter when it is often covered up.

However you should extend your skin care programme to include this area, or you will find that it ages quickly. To counteract this, use a rich moisturizing cream, and keep the area free from make up. Massage your neck with your finger tips in an upward outward motion as you apply the cream.

There are other times, too, when it is worth applying extra moisturizer:

- before and after having a bath or shower
- when you shampoo and dry your hair
- when you go out in the cold or the sun
- before you start cooking
- whenever you are likely to drink a lot of alcohol or spend time in a smoky atmosphere
- halfway through the day if your office is overheated
- before you board an aeroplane
- when you are ill, especially if you have a temperature

EXFOLIATION

Removing the dead surface cells from the skin, or exfoliating as it is properly called, is said to help the skin look fresh and glowing. This is because if the cells remain too long on the skin surface they tend to make it look dull, and may also flake and clog the sebaceous pores, leading to superficial spots and blackheads.

Exfoliation speeds up this flaking and shedding of the skin cells by removing the uppermost dead layer to reveal finer, more translucent tissue underneath. It is usually carried out once a week, or twice weekly if the skin looks at all scaly.

The skin is first cleansed thoroughly, after which a special exfoliating product is applied, and then wiped off with a rough wet facecloth. You can make your own exfoliator by combining roasted oatmeal and water to make a paste, or you can use sea salt on your facecloth, but whatever product you use you need to proceed with caution, especially if you have a dry sensitive skin. You should complete the process by applying your normal moisturizer.

The body skin also benefits from a good going over with a loofah about once a fortnight in order to boost circulation and encourage dead skin cells to flake off. Areas which need particular attention are the upper arms, thighs, buttocks, knees and elbows. After your bath apply a nourishing body lotion.

HOW TO USE A FACE MASK

A mask applied once or twice a week (depending on skin type - see chart) helps to improve the circulation, and draws out any hidden dirt and toxins. Steaming has a similar effect, but should be avoided by those with sensitive skins, or a tendency to thread veins. You will find some suggestions for suitable face masks in Chapter 11.

Before you apply a mask, cleanse your face, and apply a toner as you would normally. Put the mask on all over your face, but avoid the eye area. Most masks give the best results if they are left on for a period of time (usually up to twenty minutes), and you could treat this as an ideal opportunity to lie down and relax with your feet up.

Greasy skins or those prone to acne benefit from a mask that is allowed to set firm (you can also try dabbing a little on individual spots each day), but dry and sensitive skins will do better with a softer mask which is left on for the minimum length of time. Either way, you should always remove the mask when it begins to feel tight on the skin.

Remove the mask with warm water, then pat your skin dry and apply your usual toner and moisturizer. Your skin will feel wonderfully smooth and clean. A word of warning though – do not apply a mask a day or two before a special occasion, since it can sometimes draw impurities to the surface of the skin, thus marring your complexion with unwanted spots.

THE AGES OF BEAUTY

Although the basic beauty routine outlined above applies throughout one's life, the skin does have certain different stages, and it helps if one is aware of these.

Children, for instance, rarely have any skin problems if they are eating a healthy balanced diet, and it should be sufficient to wash their faces twice a day with a very mild soap and to otherwise leave alone. However, their skin should be protected from the sun, and from extremely cold weather.

As a child begins to approach *puberty* so the skin begins to show signs of increased oil gland activity, and this is the time to encourage a child (girls of this age will take little persuasion) to take a bit more trouble over cleansing. Rubbing the skin with a face cloth helps to keep the pores open (but do make sure the cloth is kept scrupulously clean).

With the onset of puberty and the *teenage years* the rising hormone levels affect the skin, which becomes increasingly oily with enlarged pores. This is the age at which acne is particularly prevalent (see page 46), and to counteract the extra oiliness skin should be kept scrupulously clean using a good cleanser, followed by an astringent, and a light moisturizer applied to any dry areas during the day. This skin care routine should be continued on through the *twenties*, when hormone levels are still high, and when oil and sweat glands may be even more active than they were during the teens.

Once a woman enters her *thirties* the skin is beginning to show early signs of ageing (hopefully undetectable to any but the most observant). Fine lines begin to appear around the corners of the eyes, where the skin is at its thinnest and where there are fewer sebaceous glands than anywhere else in the body. This is followed by the appearance of "smile" lines running from the corners of the nose to the corners of the mouth, and "frown" lines down the centre of the forehead. Dryness can accentuate wrinkles, even though it does not actually cause them, so guard against this by using a good moisturizer. This will also help to offset the decreasing rate of sebum production. Between the ages of 35 and 80 the rate of cell division and replacement falls off by an amazing 50 per cent, accompanied by an increased tendency for the old cells to remain longer on the skin surface, so exfoliate regularly (see page 35).

During the *forties*, as the menopause approaches, the hormonally responsive sebaceous glands begin to shrink and produce less oil, so the skin becomes drier and prone to flaking. Now is the time to start using a rich night cream, and a heavier cleanser and moisturizer than previously.

The menopause takes its toll on the condition of the skin and hair with the gradual decrease in the production of oestrogen. Continue to use rich creams on the skin. Exfoliation is now more important than ever (twice a week if possible) to ensure the skin texture remains smooth and glowing, but because the skin is drier and more delicate, use only the mildest of lotions and avoid the more abrasive techniques.

As the skin ages the outer part becomes thicker, while the inner layer is thinner and greatly weakened because the collagen and elastin fibres have begun to twist and bind together, leading to wrinkles, sagging and loss of skin tone. Facial massage and exercises help to counteract this tendency to sagging. This is the time to use a lighter hand when applying make up to the face, since it tends to settle into the creases, accentuating every line. The complexion tone changes with age, so check that your make up colours are still suitable, and steer clear of black mascara and liner, frosted shadows and bright dramatic colours since these are all more ageing.

As you get older, so the circulation slows down and you tend to put on weight more easily. Counteract this by eating a healthy diet and by taking regular exercise (see Chapter 2).

CHOOSING AND USING MAKE UP

There is no such thing as completely natural make up, because it is impossible to make without the inclusion of some synthetic ingredients. For instance, make up must contain certain colour pigments, and those taken solely from natural sources would not do the job adequately. Natural plant colours can be used for some creams and lotions, but they do not have enough staying power for make up to be used on eyes, cheeks and lips. It is also important to include efficient preservatives in make up, since it usually takes a long time to use up.

Having said that, there are several companies now who offer a range of make up which has been manufactured without involving any cruelty to animals and which is free from animal ingredients. This in itself often means using synthetic ingredients instead, for instance cetyl alcohol in place of the now banned sperm whale oil. Such make up is also likely to contain extra natural ingredients, such as herbs, jojoba, or sesame oil.

The make up look for the 80s is soft and subtle, but it can still considerably improve or alter a woman's appearance. Make up can be used, for instance, to disguise the fact that your eyes are too deep set, or too wide apart. On the other hand, eye make up incorrectly applied can quite spoil the look of someone who would otherwise be beautiful. If you want to wear make up regularly, it might well be worth investing in a visit to a beauty salon, where you can pick up valuable tips on the right way to go about things.

Always apply make up to skin that has first been cleansed, toned and moisturized. Choose your colours with care, and keep all your make up within the same range of colours. For instance cool pink shades suit pale skins, while a warm slightly orange tint is good for a pinker skin.

Eye make up can be matched either with your eye colour or with the clothes you intend to wear.

Foundation goes on first, and this not only protects the skin from pollution but also helps keep moisture in. It also hides any blemishes and gives a more even skin tone. Choose a colour as close as possible to your natural skin tone (test on the back of your hand before buying). Use a thin liquid foundation if your skin is oily, or a richer oil-based one if your skin is dry. Apply with a damp sponge.

Powder is applied on top of foundation to help set it and to prevent any shiny oily patches from showing through. Choose a loose powder for oily skins, or a block powder for a dry skin.

A blusher if carefully applied can be used to alter the natural shape of the face as well as to add colour. To find

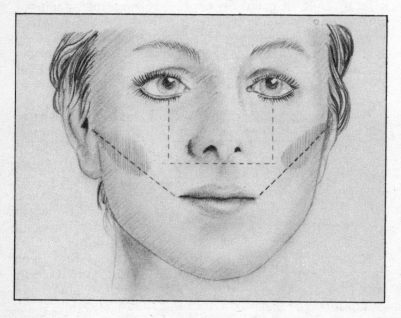

Figure 1

out the right place to apply blusher to your cheeks, imagine a line drawn from your earhole to the corner of your mouth. The blusher should be applied along that imaginary line, but no further in than the middle of the eye and no further down than below the level of the nose. The edges must be softened with a cosmetic sponge. Apply a cream blusher with your finger tips, or a powder blusher with a cosmetic brush. (See Fig. 1).

Eye shadows come in powders, creams or sticks, but if your eyelids are at all dry, you will find that a powder stays in place longest. Start by putting a foundation of a white or beige shadow all over the lid, then apply your chosen colour from the inner corner of the eye about a third of the way along, from the eyebrow and down over the lid.

Next comes the eye pencil, which is used to make the eyes look larger and more dramatic. Black is very harsh for any but those with a very dark complexion, so either match your eyeliner to your eye colour or choose a softer shade like brown or grey. Draw a thin line underneath the bottom lashes, and then apply a small triangle of eyeliner on the lid at the outer corner of the eye. Soften the edges with a sponge tip applicator.

The second application of eyeshadow (in a slightly paler

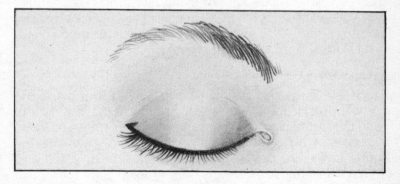

Figure 2

shade than the first) then goes on over this triangle and the base colour, from the outer corner of the eye to the mid eyebrow, again from the eyebrow down. This means that the centre part is the pale base colour only—which sounds very strange but looks most effective if applied properly. Again, soften the edges of the powder, and if you like draw another thin line of eyeliner from the centre of the lid to the outer corner. (See Fig. 2).

Mascara should be applied in several thin coats to prevent clogging the lashes, and as with eyeliner a colour like brown or navy is softer than black. Coat both the top and bottom of the upper lashes, brushing down from the top and then upwards. Use downward strokes for the lower lashes, and allow each coat to dry before applying another one. A non-waterproof mascara is easiest to remove and least harmful to the eyes. To thicken your lashes, try an application of talcum powder or face powder in between coats of mascara. After the final coat of mascara, use a fine dry brush to gently separate the lashes.

Lip colour is best applied with a special lip brush. In this way you can first draw a line round the outer contours of your lips, and then fill in the middle. If you find that your lipstick tends to run, try applying a coat of lipstick, blotting the lips with a tissue and applying a second coat.

If you want to achieve a special make up look for the evening, follow the same basic principles outlined above, but choose more dramatic colours.

MUSCLE TONE

Facial exercises also have a part to play in improving the complexion, since they serve to stimulate the circulation, tone the muscles, and discourage wrinkle formation. These exercises, which really involve little more than making funny faces, are best practised in seclusion or you'll find yourself getting some very strange looks!

At any time you should try not to tense your facial

muscles, since this not only looks unsightly but encourages wrinkles. You'll probably find that whenever you are under stress you tend to tense up certain muscles in your face, and it will take a conscious effort to break this habit.

Here are a few simple face exercises, which can be practised whenever you have a few spare minutes:

1. Open your eyes as wide as you can and count to five.
2. Purse your lips together as if you were going to whistle. Follow this by opening your mouth as wide as you can.
3. Puff out your cheeks as far as you can and count to ten. Expel air rapidly.
4. A good exercise for the neck, which also helps aching shoulders, is to rotate your head all the way round in a circle, stretching your neck as much as possible. Do this three times in each direction.
5. Raise your eyebrows as high as you can, and hold for a count of six.

CARING FOR YOUR BODY

So far we have concentrated on caring for the face, but having given it all this attention, it is important not to neglect the rest of your body.

To delay the ageing process, it is important to keep the skin all over the body well moisturized. The simplest way to do this is to add a moisturizing oil or lotion to your bath water, the oil being preferable for drier skins, although it does tend to leave the bath in rather a mess. If you suffer from really dry skin, you should rub in a moisturizing body lotion after your bath. Do this while your skin is still warm and slightly damp, so that the moisturizer soaks really well into the skin. This treatment is also to be recommended when you return, sun tanned but dry-skinned, from a holiday.

BATH PREPARATIONS

You can alter the nature of your bath by the ingredients you add to it, but there is no need to spend a lot of money on expensive bath preparations. A good bath oil, for instance, can be made by mixing a cupful of vegetable oil with a teaspoonful of herbal shampoo. Add a few drops of perfume if you like, and beat or blend the ingredients until well mixed. Use about four tablespoonsful of this mixture for each bath.

Bran or oatmeal tied in a muslin cloth and added to the bathwater softens and smoothes the skin. Don't try adding it loose to the bath, though, or you'll have an awful job scraping all the bits off your skin! Use one tablespoonful for a bath. You can also use the cloth as a wash cloth to rub off any rough skin, especially on the heels, knees, elbows, thighs or upper arms. These are areas to pay special attention to, since they can easily become dry and develop the appearance of orange peel. Rub them with a rough cloth or friction mitt whenever you have a bath, and add plenty of moisturizer after drying.

A spoonful of honey added to the bathwater is said to relax and aid sleep, while a bagful of herbs adds a luxurious scent to the water. To soothe aching muscles, soften the skin, and relieve any itchiness, add a cupful of cider vinegar to your bath, and let yourself soak for 15 to 20 minutes. (The smell will soon wear off!). You'll also find other bathtime ideas in Chapter 10.

Remember not to have the water too hot when bathing—75–80°F is quite hot enough. If you can stand the shock, a cold bath or shower is very invigorating, and helps to stimulate the circulation. After your bath, gently pat and rub yourself dry, before applying your body lotion, talcum powder and deodorant.

Deodorants are in fact a fairly recent invention, and in the early part of the century women had to resort to a dusting with talcum powder to stop themselves 'glowing'!

Cream deodorants started to become popular in the 1920s and 30s, but it was not until the 1950s that the first roll on and stick deodorants appeared, followed shortly afterwards by aerosols.

A deodorant does not prevent the body sweating, but its antiseptic ingredients act on the sweat to prevent it going rancid. Antiperspirants, on the other hand, contain a special ingredient which actually causes the pores to contract and so decreases the amount of perspiration. Traditionally this ingredient is aluminium salt, and although this has been used for years, it is by no means a natural product. Some people in fact are allergic to it, and there have also been scares about possible carcinogenic (cancer inducing) properties. Some antiperspirants today may contain zirconium in place of the aluminium salts, and this tends to be less irritating to the skin. Men's deodorants and antiperspirants are made in the same way, but contain extra active ingredients.

Sweating is, of course, a natural body function acting both as a cooling system and a means of excreting toxins. The amount we sweat varies from one person to the next, and is largely determined by heredity. The least harmful way of coping with sweat is to wash regularly, since it is not the sweat itself that smells, but the bacteria which attack it on the skin.

Antiperspirants sold in the health food shop are likely to have a formula similar to more commercial ones, although they may also contain other natural ingredients. Deodorants, on the other hand, are likely to be more natural. One well known brand, from America for instance, uses propylene glycol (derived from petroleum), witchhazel, aloe vera gel, water, oat flour (to condition the skin), xanthan gum (from vegetable sources), chamomile extract and coriander oil.

CHAPTER FOUR

BEAUTY PROBLEMS

No matter how scrupulously you care for your appearance, there is almost bound to be a time when you are faced with a beauty problem of one sort or another. If it is like most beauty problems, it will probably crop up just when you least want it, like that annoying spot which appears on the very day that you have an important engagement.

Armed with the right information, however, most of the common problems can be overcome with care and perseverance. This chapter sets out some of the more frequent problems, and tells you how to cope with them. You'll also find that the general chapters on caring for your hair/skin/eyes, etc., contain information relevant to such problems as greasy skin or dry hair, so it is worth referring to these too.

ACNE
This is most common during adolescent years, when it is caused at least in part by a hormone imbalance. Controversy still exists as to the causes of acne, but some experts attribute this complaint to an excessive intake of animal fats and of chocolate in particular (which is, of course, high in both fat and sugar). As most of us know to our cost, spots or blackheads can appear at any stage of life. Spots occur when an excess of oil is secreted by the sebaceous glands, and as it rises to the surface of the skin its exit is blocked by dirt. This causes the sebum to harden and fester, resulting in a spot. Where the tip of this comes into contact with the air it is oxidized and turns black, giving the characteristic blackhead.

First and foremost with acne, the skin must be kept scrupulously clean. The skin should be cleansed two or three times each day using a medicated cleanser, followed by a medicated or pure soap if your skin is also very greasy. Resist the temptation to squeeze spots and blackheads, and touch the infected area as little as possible, ensuring that your hands are clean to prevent the spread of infection. After cleansing apply an astringent, followed by a light liquid moisturizer used very sparingly to counteract any tendency to flakiness. Avoid wearing make up whenever possible.

Orthodox medicine's answer to acne is to treat the condition with antibiotics such as tetracycline, and although this causes noticeable improvement in as many as 75 per cent of cases, such results are only likely to be temporary, since the acne is being suppressed rather than cured. The antibiotic kills the bacteria inhabiting the spots, but it does nothing to affect the underlying causes of the blocked pores. Also the bacteria gradually become resistant to the antibiotics, and when medication is then stopped the condition deteriorates further. Some people suffer toxic or allergic reactions to antibiotics, and these drugs also encourage yeast infections (candida albicans) which can give rise to recurrent attacks of thrush and cystitis.

You should also pay attention to your diet, avoiding fried, starchy or refined foods, chocolate, coffee, carbonated drinks and alcohol. Eat as much fresh fruit and vegetables as you can. A supplement of the B vitamin complex helps to reduce oily skin, with riboflavin, niacin and pyridoxine being of particular benefit. Vitamin C has also proved helpful in treating acne, as have high doses of vitamin A.

The mineral zinc also helps many acne sufferers, and without any unpleasant side effects. This was discovered accidentally at a Swedish hospital, and has since been used with great success in Sweden, Denmark and Norway. Clinical trials lasting three months and involving teenagers and young adults have shown very encouraging results, with many patients seeing an improvement within four weeks, and the majority finding their acne almost or completely healed by the end of the 12 week period. Deficiencies of zinc are in fact increasingly common in both America and many European countries, with intakes averaging between 5 and 7 mg daily, far below the normal minimum daily requirement of 15–20 mg. The assimilation of zinc is assisted by the presence of sufficient calcium, and this mineral is also important to acne sufferers, since it helps maintain the correct acid/alkaline balance of the skin.

Another supplement which is often helpful in cases of acne is lecithin. This is derived from soya beans and acts as an emulsifier in the body, i.e., it helps to break down and disperse fats. Take two tablespoonsful of lecithin granules, or six capsules daily. You should also be sure to get plenty of sleep, exercise and fresh air to improve your circulation, and increase the flow of blood to the skin surface.

A face mask two or three times a week helps to heal and draw blemishes to the surface, while at the same time stimulating the circulation and minimizing any open pores. Use a steam facial first, following the instructions in the chart on page 60, since this helps to open the pores. Then apply a mask of natural yogurt, or a mixture of honey and wheat germ, remembering to avoid the delicate eye area. After about twenty minutes, rinse the mask off with warm water, then apply your usual astringent and moisturizer.

AGE SPOTS

This is the unflattering name given to the brown spots which sometimes appear on the backs of the hands. These are attributed to a lack of vitamins E, C and B, so it could be beneficial to take a natural supplement of these vitamins.

Bleaching sometimes helps the spots to disappear—try equal parts of cider vinegar, distilled water and milk, or equal parts of lemon juice and rosewater. Pat on to the affected area, and leave on for between fifteen minutes and several hours. Wash off with tepid water, pat dry, and apply an astringent followed by a rich moisturizing cream.

DANDRUFF

This is usually one of two different types: dry or oily. The presence of either form suggests an imbalance in the body, often due to faulty diet. Dry dandruff is usually concentrated around the ears and the hair line, and can be very itchy. Many factors are thought to contribute to dandruff, such as emotional tension, poor health, harsh shampoos, exposure to cold, and general tiredness.

It is important to keep the hair and scalp clean to minimize the accumulation of dead cells. Brush the hair daily to improve the circulation and remove any flakiness. Another daily habit to acquire is to massage the scalp thoroughly, using your fingertips and working systematically over the head (see instructions on page 84). Extra benefit can be achieved if you apply a herbal tonic before your daily massage. Steep a handful of herbs such as nettle or rosemary in a pint of boiling water, and leave to stand for up to three hours. Strain, and comb through your hair before massaging. This same tonic can be used as a final rinse after shampooing.

Another measure which helps to counteract dandruff is to dilute cider vinegar with an equal quantity of water, and dab this on to the hair with cotton wool in between shampooing. Cider vinegar added to the final rinsing water after shampooing also helps to disperse dandruff.

As far as diet is concerned, it is important to eat plenty of fresh raw fruit and vegetables, and to drink as much water as you can. At the same time, avoid fatty foods, sugar and refined carbohydrates.

THINNING OR FALLING HAIR

Every day we shed between 40 and 100 hairs, but in the normal way these are replaced by new growth. However, certain illnesses or stages in life can cause more hair than usual to be lost, for instance after having a baby, after surgery, during particularly stressful periods, or in middle age. Hair loss also varies according to the seasons, with the greatest losses being found over a period of a few weeks in both spring and autumn.

To minimize hair loss, check that you are eating the right foods for healthy hair (see page 81). Particularly important are the B vitamins, which are best supplied by brewer's yeast, wholemeal bread, liver, wheat germ, and wholegrains. Take a daily brewer's yeast supplement, either in the form of powder, or tablets (up to six daily).

Although you may be reluctant to touch your head for fear of aggravating the hair loss, daily massage is essential to stimulate the scalp circulation and promote new growth. Try gently pulling the hair too, but only when it is dry since any pressure on wet hair will stretch and break it. The nettle tonic recommended for dandruff can be used in conjunction with massage as a means of stimulating hair growth. If you have long hair, change the position of your parting regularly to prevent strain on the roots, which could stop the follicles from producing new hair. For the same reason, don't keep your hair tied back in a pony tail for long periods.

Always use warm as opposed to hot water for washing the hair, avoiding the use of harsh detergent shampoos. Try a soap-based one, or a mild baby shampoo instead. It is best to let your hair dry naturally, and not to use rollers of any kind. If you feel you must set your hair, tie several layers of tissues around the rollers, or use foam ones which are gentler on the hair.

Tension is also said to be a factor in hair loss, and it is the increased stresses of life today which are blamed for the fact that many women are now showing a tendency to baldness. So, learn how to relax.

FACIAL AND BODY HAIR

Facial hair is a problem encountered by many women, and is particularly common during the menopause. The hair is usually to be found above the upper lip, or on the sides of the face.

There are several methods of removing facial hair, and the one you choose depends very much on the severity of the problem. Plucking should be considered only if there are one or two stray hairs. Bleaching is suitable only for very fine, downy hair. Commercial bleaching agents are available but since these usually contain ammonia they are unsuitable for sensitive skins. You can make up your own lotion by mixing ½ cup of peroxide to a paste with fine oatmeal. Spread this thickly on to the skin and leave for 10 to 15 minutes before rinsing off with lots of warm water. Hair will become lighter after successive applications, but it is best to leave at least three days between each. You should also test the solution first on the back of your hand in case it causes an allergic reaction. Any form of bleach tends to dry the skin, so use plenty of nourishing cream afterwards.

Some depilatory creams are produced specifically for facial hair, but as with the bleach, do an allergy test before embarking. This initial testing is particularly important when using depilatory products, since they are the ones most likely to cause a skin reaction. A variety of creams, lotions and foam mousses is available, and they work by means of a chemical, usually thioglycolic acid. This acid is neutralized with sodium hydroxide and calcium hydroxide, so that a normally strongly alkaline chemical is adjusted to a pH of 12–13. This is still considerably more alkaline than the skin which has a pH of 6.5. The acid in the product breaks up cystine, a major amino acid in the hair, so that the hair becomes very brittle and breaks easily when the product is wiped off the skin. Because the chemical actually penetrates just below the skin's surface, breaking into the hair shaft, the new hair which grows back looks completely natural. The only permanent method of removing hair is electrolysis, a method in which the hair root is cauterized by giving it a tiny electric shock. The success of this treatment depends on the skill of the operator, so always ensure that a reputable salon is chosen. Unskilled electrolysis could result in nasty scarring.

A variety of methods is available for those women who need to remove unsightly hairs from their legs. Shaving is one method that is quick and easy, but its disadvantage is that the new hair growth tends to look thicker. This is because shaving shears the hairs off at skin level, thus blunting the tips of the new hairs. It is a fallacy that hair grows back more quickly after shaving. It is advisable to use body lotion on the legs after shaving to counteract any dryness. And when it comes to shaving under the arms, avoid using a deodorant or antiperspirant (see page 45) for at least 12 hours in case of any chemical irritation (a mild talc can be used in the interim if you are concerned about body odour).

Waxing is the most natural method of removing hair, and although this can be carried out at home it is far easier to have it done at a beauty salon. Various different formulae are used, all based on natural waxes such as beeswax, with other ingredients added to make it melt easily. The wax is heated to the required temperature, spread thinly on the skin and then covered with strips of a special material, which are then pulled away, removing both hair and wax. In this treatment the hair is literally torn out, so it can be quite painful. As with facial hair, depilatory products, electrolysis or bleaching may also be used.

GREY HAIR

This is largely determined by heredity—and there is nothing you can do about that! However, premature greyness can be delayed by increasing scalp circulation, and by ensuring an abundance of certain nutrients in the diet. Tests have shown that foods rich in iodine, iron, copper, vitamins B and F can help restore colour to greying hair, but any improvements are likely to be visible only after a good few months. Pantothenic acid, PABA (*P*-aminobenzoic acid) and folic acid are the three B vitamins said to restore colour. If you want to try a treatment, said by one American doctor to have a 70 per cent success rate, take a daily supplement of 100mg PABA, 30mg calcium pantothenate, and 2 grammes of choline. Since these are all present in brewer's yeast, this may be the simplest way to supplement.

EYE WRINKLES

As you will read in the chapter on eyes, the skin in this area is so delicate that it is one of the first to wrinkle, especially if maltreated. You should follow the general advice given in that chapter, but in addition try using an eye cream containing vitamin E (such as that on page 132). This vitamin is said to delay and minimize wrinkles if used consistently over a period of time, but remember to apply the cream correctly (see page 97), or you will simply aggravate the problem.

THREAD VEINS

These are particularly common in those with a dry or sensitive skin. Once acquired they are difficult to eradicate, but you can help prevent them from growing worse by increasing your daily vitamin C intake (i.e., plenty of fresh raw fruit and vegetables, especially citrus fruits, blackcurrants, and green peppers). This is because these broken veins are believed to be caused by lack of vitamin C in the diet.

Try to avoid tea, coffee and alcohol, each of which aggravates the condition. Drink herb teas instead. You can make these yourself in the same way that you would make ordinary tea, using 1 teaspoonful dried or 3 teaspoonsful fresh herb per person, plus one for the pot. Pour on boiling water and leave to stand for 5 minutes before drinking. Coltsfoot is particularly suitable.

It is important to avoid extremes of temperature. Use only warm water when washing, and protect the skin with a moisturizer before venturing out in cold or hot weather. Steam facials should also be avoided.

In severe cases thread veins can be treated by electrolysis, which is used to dry up the tiny veins. There is nothing this treatment can do to prevent fresh outbreaks elsewhere though. A marigold lotion, made from the flowers infused in boiling water (follow the instructions for nettle tonic on page 49), can help if patted on to the affected area each day after cleansing. It is also worth rubbing the face with the inside peel of citrus fruit. Thread veins can now be treated by laser beam, which is a painless and effective way of cauterizing the veins, but this treatment is not widely available, and is very expensive.

PROBLEM NAILS

General advice on caring for your nails is given on page 112, but there are several problems which are commonly experienced in this area, as follows:

● **White spots on the nails**. These suggest a diet too low in zinc, calcium or vitamin B6. Increase your intake of foods rich in these nutrients, such as nuts, cheese, wholegrains, dried fruits and green vegetables.

● **Hangnails.** These torn shreds of skin beside the nails are usually the result of dryness, so keep applying a rich moisturizer, and resist the temptation to cut them.

● **Slow growing nails.** Make sure your diet contains

sufficient protein and vitamin E. A supplement of oil of evening primrose may help. Try some simple exercises to stimulate circulation and growth, such as drumming the nails gently on a table. Buffing the nails (see page 113) also assists growth.

● **Splitting nails.** It may be worth taking a supplement of the B complex vitamins, as well as a multimineral supplement. Avoid sawing at the nails when shaping them, and have them unprotected in water as little as possible.

● **Brittle nails.** Keep free from varnish and remover whenever possible, and increase your intake of the B vitamins.

● **Ridged nails.** These ridges are sometimes formed at times of acute illness, but they can also suggest a chronically poor state of health. Get plenty of vitamins A, B and D.

● **Soft nails.** Avoid hot water and all detergents including soap (try one of the soapless cleansers). Ensure your diet is high in vitamins and minerals. A traditional remedy is to drink a tablespoonful of gelatine, mixed into water or juice and drunk straight away, once a day.

● **Nail biting.** Often a sign of stress, so take more B vitamins to counteract this and try to reduce your stress levels.

SENSITIVITY TO COSMETICS

It is extremely rare for somebody to be *allergic* to cosmetics, but many people suffer from sensitivity, usually to a group of substances rather than to one particular component, which makes it very difficult to know which products are affecting you adversely. Those most likely to suffer from sensitivity are people with pale skins, red or fair hair, dry skin, or those who have a tendency towards asthma, hayfever, eczema, or who burn easily in the sun. Signs of sensitivity are frequent dry, red, itchy patches on the skin of the face, neck or body.

The situation is further complicated in that it is quite possible to suddenly become sensitive to a product you have been using for years. However, it may help to identify the offending product by asking yourself the following questions:

- Have I recently tried a new product, or has my usual product undergone a change in formulation?
- Is the condition restricted to a specific area? (The area affected may not relate to where the product was applied!)
- Is the condition worse at some times and better at others, for instance after washing my hair, or applying perfume?

If you have still not come up with an answer, the only other way is to embark on a gradual process of elimination, cutting out one product at a time until you track down the one that is causing the problem.

There are certain items which are recognized as being common sensitizers, and in America ingredients-listing helps to reveal the presence of these. Under EEC regulations, which are expected to be introduced in the United Kingdom, a product would have to show whether one or more of these potential sensitizers had been included.

The following are particularly likely to cause trouble:

- aluminium salts, found in antiperspirants. Sensitivities and irritation are common, particularly if skin is already sore, or newly shaved.
- perfumes, the most common of all sensitizers, especially those with a chemical rather than a natural base. If you suspect perfumes, look for simple, unscented products instead. As mentioned on page 134, unless a product states that it is unperfumed, it will contain some scent.
- parabens, a group of preservatives used in low concentration in many cosmetic and medicinal preparations. Other preservatives which may also cause trouble are quaternium 15, imidazolidiny urea, and formaldehyde. The latter is used in high concentration in nail hardening products, and its use may cause discoloura-

tion or separation of the nails.

- frosted eyeshadow or lipsticks contain an ingredient which makes them irridescent but which may also cause irritation.
- lanolin, although a natural product, can upset some users, producing a dry scaly rash, often with severe inflammation. Products described as 'superfatted' or 'moisturizing' may well contain lanolin. Look for creams containing petrolatum instead.
- paraphenylenediamine, an ingredient of permanent hair dyes, hence the importance of doing a patch test first (see page 90).
- aerosol products can cause irritation if you are prone to sensitivity, as can the chemicals in the spray.
- sun tan products may contain fragrances that affect some skins adversely, and because they tend to be worn in intense heat, any harmful reaction may be accentuated.
- nail polish can cause irritation, but is more likely to be apparent on the face than the hands, which can be very misleading.

DRY SKIN

An excessively dry skin can be caused either by external or internal factors. The sun is the skin's number one arch enemy and dehydrator. Prolonged exposure to the sun without adequate protection, even at an early age, triggers off dehydration, destroys the skin's elastin and collagen fibres, and causes it to thicken up as a defence mechanism. The result is a prematurely lined, dry skin such as is often seen among people living in hot climates.

Other extremes of weather, cold and wind, air conditioning, central heating and too much soap on the skin can all cause dry skin by moisture evaporation. Smoking, too, is another common cause of dry skin.

Internal causes leading to dry skin are hormonal imbalances (for instance in pregnancy or at the menopause), illness, stress, severe dieting, or surgery. If your skin fails to respond to your usual moisturizer, or if it is dry regardless of weather or external conditions, then it is likely that the cause is internal. In this case the first step is to make sure the diet contains plenty of protein, especially from non-animal sources. The diet also needs to contain ample fat, and you can ensure this by using a teaspoonful each day (for instance in salad dressings) of a polyunsaturated oil such as safflower or sunflower. A B complex vitamin should also prove helpful. Make sure, too, to drink plenty of fluids (preferably mineral waters), and eat lots of green vegetables for their mineral and fluid content.

As far as external care of dry skin is concerned, it is a question of keeping the natural moisture in and preventing excessive moisture loss. This means always protecting the skin from the elements by wearing a light, easily absorbed cream during the day, and a thicker richer one at night. If these are applied while the skin is still slightly damp absorption rate will be improved.

A cleansing cream and a light toner are best when it comes to cleansing a dry skin, but if you prefer to use water choose one of the soapless cleansing bars in place of soap since these do not upset the natural pH level of the skin. If you are simply troubled with patches of dry flaky skin on an otherwise normal or oily skin, then you need to treat each area separately.

If your skin is very badly dried out then professional treatment from an aromatherapist will undoubtedly help. You can also prepare your own treatment by blending 7 drops of geranium oil with 15 of sandalwood oil and 3 of rose oil and 50 ml. of vegetable oil. First cleanse the skin, leaving it slightly damp, then pat the oil on all over. Lean over a basin of steaming water or lie in the bath to assist penetration. If you can, leave the oil on overnight and then remove it the following morning with a gentle face tonic.

For skin that is dry all over, try adding a few drops of oil to your bathwater, but take care because this does make the bath slippery. After your bath, massage in plenty of body lotion.

Current research into dehydration and ageing has found that using cosmetics which are predominantly alkaline destroys the skin's natural acid barrier and eventually retards its renewal mechanism. Dryness, wrinkles and sensitivity result, and of course the skin becomes more vulnerable to external aggravation. Overzealous and harsh cleansing, hard and very hot water, alcohol-based products and detergents can also progressively strip the skin's pH factor.

YOUR SKIN CARE CHART

Skin Type	How to Recognize	Cleanse	Tone
Normal	Smooth, soft and fine textured. The occasional spot but no real problems. In fact it's a very rare skin type.	Light cleansing cream, or a rinse-off cleanser with water. Eye make up remover for delicate eye area.	Light skin tonic.
Greasy	Face quickly becomes shiny. Tissue held to skin looks greasy. Prone to open pores and blemishes, especially around nose.	2-3 times daily use a medicated cleanser or a rinse-off cleanser.	Apply astringent, paying particular attention to greasiest areas like sides of nose, chin and forehead.
Dry	Flaky and dull, especially round eyes and on cheeks. Feels taut after using soap, and becomes red and sore in cold weather.	Massage in rich cleansing cream, and wipe off with cotton wool. Avoid using tap water – if necessary use creamy face wash and mineral water once a day.	Very gentle toner, avoiding upper cheeks. Dilute toner if skin is very dry.
Combi-nation	A greasy panel down centre of face, with dryish areas on cheeks and around eyes.	Use a light cream, especially on greasy areas. Follow this with a rinse-off cleanser or soap on greasy areas only.	Light toning lotion, followed by astringent on greasy areas.

Moisturize	Special Treatment	Diet
Light liquid moisturizer night and morning. A light eye cream at night. Light throat cream.	Weekly mask or light steam facial. Use the latter only if no thread veins. Add a handful of rosemary or chamomile to 1 pt. (550ml) boiling water. Put face about 12 inches above bowl, cover head, and remain for 5 minutes. Finish with toner and moisturizer.	Plenty of fresh raw fruit and vegetables, protein and wholegrains.
A light liquid moisturizer especially on cheeks. Eye and neck creams.	Twice a week use a mask or steam facial with rosemary or sage. Finish with an astringent.	Avoid fatty or fried food, chocolate, tea, coffee, and alcohol. Eat plenty of green vegetables.
Light moisturizer during the day, with a rich nourishing cream at night. Use this on neck as well. Apply eye cream each night too.	Moisturizing facial once weekly, e.g. honey, avocado or egg yolk. Leave on for up to 20 minutes, then wipe off, tone and moisturize.	Include unsaturated fats in the form of vegetable oils and nuts. Get plenty of vitamins A, B complex, C and E.
Liquid moisturizer all over face, followed by rich nourishing cream on dry areas.	Once a week face mask, using one of the suggestions for dry skin on cheeks, and egg white and lemon juice on greasy centre panel.	As for normal skin, but restrict greasy foods.

CHAPTER FIVE

A SENSIBLE APPROACH TO SLIMMING

Obesity and beauty definitely don't go together. It's hard to look beautiful when you're bulging in all the wrong places, although it's not just your face and figure which are affected when you are carrying excess weight. Your self-confidence suffers a severe blow too – and pride in your appearance plays an important part in being beautiful.

If you are overweight you are also placing an extra strain on your heart, and as a result you run an increased risk of falling prey to such severe ailments as coronary heart disease, high blood pressure or diabetes.

Getting your figure in trim is therefore one of the first steps to take, for the sake of both your looks and your health. You need not think that you have to be wafer thin to be beautiful. In recent years we have become diet crazy (hardly surprising, perhaps, when it is estimated that one in five adults in Britain is overweight), and there must be almost as many diets as there are overweight people.

Some of these diets are so severe and extreme that they are likely to be more detrimental to your health than being overweight. Crash diets which severely restrict food intake or exclude all but one or two food items are not to be recommended, however serious your obesity problem. Not only is your health likely to suffer, but if you do succeed in adhering to such a diet and losing weight, you are likely to put many of those lost pounds back on again once you resume your normal eating habits.

There is a risk with most slimming diets that in cutting down on the amount of food you eat, you are also drastically reducing your intake of vital nutrients. When this happens you are likely to suffer from the tiredness and irritability so familiar to slimmers. The only sensible way to lose weight (and to maintain that weight loss) is to follow a carefully balanced diet which makes up in quality for what you lose in quantity.

WHOLEFOODS

This is where wholefoods come into their own. Because they retain a higher proportion of nutrients than refined foods, you are getting more goodness from the food you eat. Wholefoods not only supply more vitamins and minerals than refined foods; their natural roughage also aids the digestion, and makes the foods more satisfying so that you need to eat less. Those following a high fibre diet have also been shown to absorb approximately ten per cent fewer calories from their food than those on a low fibre diet.

Wholefoods are not specifically slimming foods, but their extra nutritional value means that you stay happy and healthy while you slim. A wholefood diet also includes plenty of fresh fruit and vegetables, which add extra variety and goodness but very few calories. Readjusting your eating habits along wholefood lines should not be regarded as a temporary measure though. Eating the wholefood way will help you to stay slim and healthy even when you have reached your ideal weight.

Using the calorie chart and food list included in this chapter, you can work out a wholefood diet to suit yourself, bearing in mind that to achieve an appreciable weight loss, women should follow a 1000 calorie diet, and men a 1500 calorie diet. For those who prefer to follow a more rigid diet plan, a seven day wholefood diet is also included. This was devised by *Slimming Naturally*, a magazine catering for those who want to lose weight and stay healthy.

Whatever diet you choose, the following points are

worth bearing in mind while you are slimming:

Cut down the amount of fat you eat to about 1 oz. (25g) a day. Do not totally exclude fat from your diet or your skin and hair will pay the penalty. Ideally, the fat you use should be in the form of unsaturated vegetable oil or margarine, but don't on any account use these for frying or your calorie count will go shooting up.

Keep your fluid intake to a minimum, since drinking excess fluid can aggravate problems of overweight by causing fluid retention. Restrict tea and coffee to two cups a day or, better still, cut them out completely. Cut right back as well on your alcohol intake while slimming. Herb teas have no calories at all (provided you add no sweetening), and some are useful to slimmers since they are both diaphoretic (promoting sweating) and diuretic. Choose peppermint, mace, rosehip or dandelion. Lemon juice also acts as a diuretic, and, as can be seen from the seven day diet, can be taken for this purpose first thing in the morning with hot water. Having something to drink half an hour before a meal also helps to take the edge off your appetite.

Use skim milk in place of whole milk for drinks and cooking. It's much lower in calories.

If you must eat between meals, choose raw fruit or vegetables from the free list.

Cook all food carefully to retain maximum nutrient content, without increasing the calories. This means eating vegetables raw, or lightly boiled or steamed. Grill meat wherever possible, and pour away the cooking juices when roasting since these are high in fat.

Watch out for nutritious but high calorie foods such as nuts, hard cheeses, commercial fruit yogurt, and avocado pears.

Include lots of salads in your diet (they are low in calories and a good source of vitamins and minerals), but avoid high calorie dressings. Instead, try one of the following: half a carton of natural yogurt with the juice of half a lemon, and a dash of honey and mustard; large spoonful of milk powder, mixed with a spoonful each of cider vinegar and lemon juice (add a spoonful of curry powder for spicy flavour); half a cupful of tomato juice with the juice of half a lemon and a teaspoon of chopped onion, chives or garlic.

Unfortunately, no easy, painless way of losing weight has yet been discovered. Whatever diet or slimming aids you use, it's still a question of will power – without it, you're fighting a losing battle! Any diet will be far more successful if you accompany it with a regular exercise programme (see page 20), since this speeds up the metabolism, and thereby the rate at which calories are used up. Studies have shown that many overweight people actually eat less than average, but are overweight because they take too little exercise. Even an extra 30 minutes of brisk walking each day could make the difference between success and failure where dieting is concerned.

There are also some foods which can be included in a wholefood diet to speed your weight loss, and to keep you in good health while you are slimming.

THE WONDER COMBINATION –
Lecithin/Cider Vinegar/Kelp/Vitamin B6

Top of this list must come four health food ingredients which, when taken in combination, have been found by slimmers to speed up weight loss. Of course, these foods will not lead to loss of weight on their own, but must be taken in conjunction with a low calorie diet.

The Lecithin/Cider Vinegar/Kelp/Vitamin B6 low calorie diet was first discovered by an American journalist called Mary Ann Crenshaw. She labelled the four special in-gredients 'fat fighters' and she introduced the diet to readers of her book *The Natural Way to Super Beauty*, published in America in 1974. As a result, dieters on both sides of the Atlantic were soon following her example.

Indeed, the diet has become so popular that manufacturers are now producing slimming capsules which
combine all these four elements in the correct proportions
in an easy-to-take form. Such capsules are readily available
from health food shops, and they are proving to be a
continuing best seller.

It was whilst researching nutritional theory and ex-
perimenting with strict 1000 calorie diets that Mary Ann
Crenshaw discovered that, for her, these four 'fat fighters'
worked wonders. She says in her book that after using
them in her low-calorie regimen for two weeks she lost a
full 12 lb in weight, and she also found that her new diet
worked just as well on her friends.

Consistent with what is said above, she emphasizes in her
book that her Lecithin/Cider Vinegar/Kelp/Vitamin B6
formula is not a miracle slim system by itself. Your diet is the
important thing if you wish to lose weight and stay slim, but
as she says: ' . . . my four little friends sure did make things
easier. And quicker, which is the best part of all.' It is good
to know, too, that these four ingredients are not drugs but
foods.

Mary Ann Crenshaw worked out her diet on the basis of
the following theories:

Lecithin is present in every cell in the human body, and it
also occurs naturally in egg yolks, some vegetable oils and
soya beans. Lecithin acts as an emulsifier, which means that
it breaks up fat and so helps to prevent it accumulating in
the body. It also acts as a natural diuretic, and is one of the
best sources of two-hard-to-get B vitamins, choline and
inositol, both of which are important to hair health. As a
food supplement, lecithin is usually derived from soya
beans and is available in either granular or capsule form.
Mary Ann Crenshaw took one to two tablespoonsful of
lecithin granules daily on her diet, this amount being
equivalent to six British teaspoonsful.

Cider Vinegar is a rich source of many of the minerals,

and appears to have a regulating effect on the body metabolism. It has been credited with the ability to relieve a wide variety of ailments, especially arthritis and rheumatism, and throat and bronchial complaints. Mary Ann Crenshaw included it in her diet as a rich source of the mineral potassium, which encourages the body to excrete excess fluid. For the purpose of slimming, take a teaspoonful of cider vinegar in a glass of water with every meal.

Kelp is the name given to a dried seaweed, which is used as a food supplement because it is one of the richest known sources of minerals, particularly iodine. This is the mineral needed by the thyroid gland, which controls the body metabolism and therefore determines how quickly food is burned up. Women are more likely to be deficient in iodine than men, and a shortage is particularly common during adolescence and youth. Mary Ann Crenshaw, who put on weight easily and knew that she had a slow metabolism, took 200 milligrammes of kelp each day.

Vitamin B6, also known as pyrodoxine, is the member of the B complex which is essential to the nervous system, and the first signs of a deficiency are irritability and depression. Women taking the Pill are especially likely to be short of this vitamin. B6 also appears to balance the levels of potassium and sodium in the body, which means that it helps counteract fluid retention. Mary Ann Crenshaw took 50 milligrammes a day.

Other wholefoods which will assist the slimmer in his or her battle against overweight include the following:

BRAN

A valuable source of roughage, and as such will ward off the constipation which is so often experienced by slimmers. The normal amount to take is up to two tablespoonsful daily, the exact amount required varying from one person to another. A teaspoonful of bran taken in liquid before meals also helps to take the edge off the appetite, so that

you are inclined to eat less. Bran, which comes in a finely
flaked form, can be added to cereals or desserts, drinks,
savoury dishes or used in baking.

WHEAT GERM
Like bran, this is removed during the manufacture of white
flour and is prized as a rich source of vitamins E, B, and A, as
well as being 28 per cent protein. Also present are
quantities of unsaturated fats and minerals. Wheat germ
can be sprinkled on cereals, mixed into casseroles, soups or
drinks, or included in baking. It also makes a good
substitute for breadcrumbs, or can be eaten alone with
milk or yogurt.

BREWER'S YEAST
Not only a rich source of protein, but also contains the B
complex vitamins, and fourteen minerals. It's an excellent
pick-me-up, and comes in the form of tablets or powder.
The strong taste of the latter is best disguised by adding it to
soups, drinks, casseroles or cereals.

SKIM MILK POWDER
As already mentioned, this is much lower in calories than
whole milk. It is also free from fat, and is a good source of
protein, calcium, and many of the B vitamins. As well as
being used as a substitute for whole milk, a spoonful of the
powder can be added to other foods to boost their nutrient
content.

THE A TO Z OF WHOLEFOOD CALORIES
All calorie amounts are approximate, and are given per
ounce of food.

Beans (cooked)	
Butter	26
Haricot	25
Lentils	27

Biscuits	
Oatcakes	100
Savoury biscuits	120–140
Sweet biscuits	120–140

Bran	
Bran cereals	90–100
Miller's bran	92

Bread	
Granary, white or brown	70–73
Wholemeal	64

Breakfast cereals	
Flaked cereals	100–110
Granola cereals	130–140
Grapenuts	100
Muesli	100–110
Oats, uncooked	112
Porridge, cooked	13
Puffed cereals	100
Wheat biscuits	100–106

Cakes	100–140

Carob flour	51

Cheese	
Cottage	30–33
Cream	232
Curd	39
Edam	90
Other hard cheeses	100–120

Cream	
Double	131
Single	62

Crispbreads	per slice
Biscottes	30–35
Starch reduced slices	21–24
Primula Rye	17
Kelloggs Scanda Brod brown	32
Scanda Crisp	19
Ryvita	26
Rye King	28
brown	35

Dried Fruit	
Apple rings	71
Apricots	52
Currants	69
Dates	70
Figs	61
Prunes	46
Seeded raisins	80
Sultanas	71

Eggs	46

Fats and Oils	
Butter and margarine	226
Oils	262

Fish	
Oily (tuna, herring, mackerel, sardine)	65–85
Salmon, tinned	36
Shellfish	30
White fish	18–30

Flour and Grains

Uncooked wholegrains, and the flours into which they are ground range from	95–105

Fruit, fresh

Apples, grapes, cherries	14
Avocado pear	25
Banana	22
Grapefruit, melon, soft fruit	6
Lemons, gooseberries	4
Oranges, peaches	10
Pear, pineapple, plum	12
Tangerines, apricots	8

Fruit bars (per bar)	90–160

Ice Cream	50

Juices, unsweetened

Apple	10
Carrot, grapefruit, orange, lemon	12
Grape	19
Pineapple	16
Tomato, vegetable	6

Meat, fresh (lean only)

Beef	49
Chicken, veal	31
Duck, rabbit	42
Kidney (raw, lamb's)	28
Lamb, turkey	40
Liver	38
Minced beef	80
Pork	54

Milk

Buttermilk	11
Dried powder (made up)	10
Evaporated	49
Soya, liquid	10
Whole, liquid	19
Semi-skimmed	14
Skimmed	10

Nuts, shelled

Almonds	164
Brazil	180
Cashew, coconut	178
Chestnut	49
Hazel	108
Peanuts	166
Walnuts	151
Chopped, mixed	148
Mixed nuts and raisins	109
Peanut butter	180

Nutmeats

Granose Nutbrawn	37
Meatless Steaks	36
Nutmeat	57
Nuttolene	87
Prewett's Brazilia Mix	117
Rissol-nut	129
Sausalatas	36

Pasta, cooked	32

Salad dressings

Mayonnaise	202
Salad cream	108

Seeds, shelled
Linseed, sunflower	170
Pumpkin	155
Sesame	161

Sugar and sweeteners
Black treacle	75
Honey	82-90
Jam	80
Molasses	73
All sugars	112

Vegetables, fresh
Aubergine (raw), green beans, broccoli, spinach (raw), courgette (raw), watercress, radish	4
Broad beans, beetroot	13
Chicory, cucumber, lettuce	3
Carrots, onions, swedes, turnips	6
Cauliflower, cabbage, spring greens, bean sprouts, asparagus	8
Leeks	9
Mushrooms (raw),	2
Parsnips	14
Peas	20
Peppers	10
Brussels sprouts	24
Potatoes, boiled	23
Sweetcorn	28
Tomatoes, fresh	4
canned	43

Wheat germ	100

Yogurt
Low fat, unflavoured	12–16
Fruit flavoured	22

THE SEVEN DAY WHOLEFOOD DIET

Free list	Permitted in small amounts	Occasional treat
Fresh fruit:	*Fresh raw vegetables:*	*Seeds:*
Grapefruit		Linseed 170
Soft fruit,	Peas 18	Pumpkin 155
e.g., Blackberries	Potatoes 24	Sesame 161
Melon 6		Sunflower 170
Orange	*Fresh fruit:*	
Peaches 10	Apples	*Nuts:*
Pears	Grapes	Peanuts 166
Pineapple	Cherries 14	Cashew 178
Plums 12		Almonds 164

Free list		Permitted in small amounts		Occasional treat	
Rhubarb	2	*Meat:*			
Tangerines	8	Grilled		Sweet or	
		gammon	83	savoury	
Fresh raw		Beef (grilled)		wholewheat	
vegetables:		lean steak)	86	biscuits or	
Lettuce		Chicken (roast)	54	cakes	100–140
Mushrooms		Liver (stewed)	43		
Celery		Turkey (roast)	56	*Meat:*	
Broccoli		Veal cutlet	56	Duck (roast)	55
Green beans				Lamb (roast)	83
Spinach	2	*Meatless*		Pork (roast)	90
Swedes		*meats:*		Rissol-nut	129
Tomatoes		Meatless steak			
Turnips	4	(TVP)	36	*Fats and oils:*	
Carrots		Nutmeat	57	Butter	211
Onions	6			Margarine	211
Asparagus		*Fish:*		Oils	255
Cabbage		White fish,		Soyanutta	266
Cauliflower		e.g., cod	20		
Greens	8	Salmon		*Sugar and*	
Broad Beans		(tinned)	36	*sweeteners:*	
Beetroot		Shellfish	30 (av)	all sugar	
Parsnips	13	Oily fish, e.g.,		including	
		tuna,		Fructose	12
		mackerel,		Molasses	73
Fruit juices:		herring,			
Apple	10	sardine	65–70	*Others:*	
Grape	19			Mayonnaise	202
Tomato		*Cheese:*		Jams (natural)	80
Vegetable		Cottage, (low-		Chutney	20–40
(e.g., V8)	6	fat plain)	30-33	Single cream	51
Carrot	12	Hard, e.g.,		Fruit bars	90–160
Grapefruit	16	cheddar	100–110	Pasta	32
Orange	14			Granola	
Pineapple	16			cereals	130

Free list	Permitted in small amounts		Occasional treat	
	Beans, cooked:		Dry white	
Crispbreads:	Butter	26	wine	21
Primula Rye	Haricot	25	Draught bitter	9
extra thin	17	Lentils	27		
Scanda Crisp	19			
	Dried fruit:			
Bran	92	Apple rings	71		
	Apricots	54		
Yeast extract	2	Currants	72		
	Dates	74		
Herbs (for	Figs	54		
seasoning	Prunes	38		
and teas)	0	Seedless			
	raisins	94		
Fresh skimmed	Sultanas	74		
milk, or recon-				
stituted	*Cereals:*			
dried (20 fl.	Muesli base	110		
oz. in one	Porridge			
pint)	10	(made with			
yogurt	15	water and salt)	13		
	Wholegrain			
	boiled rice	95–105		
	Wholewheat			
	bread	64		
	Others:			
	Eggs	45		
	Outline low-			
	fat spread	105		
	Honey	82-90		
	Fresh whole			
	milk	19		

Figures given are calories per ounce (25g).

MENU SUGGESTIONS

Day One

	Calorie count
On rising:	
Cupful hot water and fresh lemon juice	0

Breakfast:		
4 oz. (100g) porridge (made with water)	52	
1 slice wholemeal toast with 4oz banana	163	
		215

Lunch:		
3 oz. (75g) mixed salad from any vegetables on free list	20	
2 oz. (50g) cottage cheese	60	
1 large slice wholemeal bread spread thinly with margarine	150	
1 fresh fruit, e.g., orange	40	
1 cup hot yeast extract	0	
		270

Supper:		
4 oz. (100g) any white fish wrapped in foil, with mushrooms, a little lemon juice, salt, herbs and ½ oz. (12½g) margarine	185	
3 oz. (75g) vegetables from free list	18	
4 oz. (100g) baked jacket potato	96	
1 fresh fruit, e.g., apple sliced with 1 oz. (25g) natural yogurt	55	
		354

Total calories for day:	839

Day Two

On rising:	
Cupful hot water and fresh lemon juice	0

Breakfast
Poached egg   90
Slice wholemeal toast and margarine   75
Grilled tomato   4
                                                          169

Lunch:
6 oz. (175g) salad (from free list)   40
1 oz. (25g) low fat natural yogurt as dressing   20
3 oz. (75g) sardines (drained of oil)   195
1 peach   20
                                                          275

Supper:
Vegetable soup (any on free list made with
   yeast extract stock and seasoned with
   herbs)   70
4 oz. (100g) cauliflower with cheese sauce
   made from 1 oz. cheddar and ¼ pt.
   (150ml) low fat skimmed milk, served
   with grilled tomato, and baked potato
   plus knob of butter   250
5 oz. (150g) cubed melon   30
                                                          350

Total calories for day: 794

Day Three

On rising:
Cupful hot water and fresh lemon juice   0

Breakfast:
2 oz. (50g) stewed prunes or apricots   45
4 oz. (100g) natural low fat yogurt   60
1 tablespoonful bran   18
1 slice wholemeal toast spread thinly with
   margarine   75
                                                          198

Lunch:
Salad Nicoise made with 1 hard boiled egg,
   1 tomato, 2–3 anchovy fillets, 3–4 black
   olives, 2 oz. (50g) cooked green beans,
   lemon juice and herb dressing   106
1 apple   38
1 oz. (25g) cheddar cheese   100
                                                        244

Supper:
Ratatouille made with vegetables from free
   list, and baked with 1 oz. (25g) oil   142
2 oz. (50g) roast chicken   108
1 large eating pear sliced and served with
   spicy lemon sauce made as follows:
   combine juice of one lemon with pinch
   ginger and pinch cinnamon. Heat for
   two minutes and leave to cool. Pour over
   pear and chill for ten minutes.   45
                                                        295

Total calories for day: 737

Day Four

On rising:
Cupful hot water and fresh lemon juice   0

Breakfast:
Half grapefruit   24
1 boiled egg with wholemeal bread   210
                                                        234

Lunch:
1 large baked potato filled with cottage
   cheese and chives and knob of butter   200
1 oz. (25g) grapes   14

                                                        214

Supper:
2 oz. (50g) raw mushrooms served with 3 oz.
  (75g) natural yogurt and little chopped
  raw onion   50
2 oz. (50g) liver stewed with tomatoes,
  onions, herbs, and served with 4 oz.
  (100g) broccoli   110
1 apple baked with ½ oz. (12½g) raisins   89

    249

Total calories for day: 697

Day Five:

On rising:
Cupful hot water and fresh lemon juice   0

Breakfast:
1 large egg scrambled with ½ oz. (12½g)
  butter   202
1 slice wholemeal bread and margarine   75

    277

Lunch:
4 crispbread spread with banana and date   152
2 oz. (50g) plain yogurt with 3 oz. (75g)
  raspberries   52

    204

Supper:
2 oz. (50g) boiled wholegrain rice mixed
  with 1 small pepper fried in ½
  teaspoonful oil and seasoned with herbs
  and soy sauce, topped with 1 oz. (25g)
  grated cheese   370
3 oz. (75g) blackberries   18

    388

Total calories for day: 869

Day Six

On rising:
Cup hot water and fresh lemon juice   0

Breakfast:
4 oz. (100g) porridge made with water   52
1 poached egg, 1 tomato and 1 oz. (25g)
    grilled mushrooms   104
                                                                156

Lunch:
Apple, cheese and celery salad, made with
    4 oz. (100g) cottage cheese, 2 sticks celery
    and 2 oz. (50g) apple   156
4 crispbread   35
                                                                191

Supper:
Kebabs: put alternately on skewers pepper,
    onion, tomato, mushrooms   42
Served with 2 oz. (50g) wholegrain rice   200
4 dessert plums with 1 oz. (25g) single cream   91
                                                                333

Total calories for day: 680

Day Seven

On rising:
Cupful hot water and fresh lemon juice   0

Breakfast:
As Day 3, without toast   123
                                                                123

Lunch:
1 oz. (25g) vegetable or liver pâté   97
2 slices wholemeal bread   123
3 oz. (75g) salad from free list   20
                                                                240

Supper:

Three sticks celery, braised in vegetable stock for 30 minutes	10
1 large baked potato with 1 oz. (25g) grated cheese and ½ oz. (12½g) butter	280
4 oz. (100g) mixed fruit salad from free list, with lemon juice and a little honey	60
	350

Total calories for day: 713

N.B. menus allow for 200 calories to be used on drinks.

CHAPTER SIX

HAIR CARE

If you are one of those people whose idea of hair care begins and ends with a quick shampoo once or twice a week, you have a lot to learn. Very few people give their hair the care and attention it needs – which is no doubt why it is so common to see hair that shows obvious signs of neglect. Certainly the sleek, shining locks one sees in glossy magazines seem to be a long way removed from everyday life.

Before you can begin to care for your hair, it helps to have at least a basic knowledge of its structure. The hair is composed of a protein-based substance called keratin – the same substance which forms finger- and toe-nails. Each hair consists of three layers, the central core or medulla being made up of spongy tissues which may contain some colour pigment. This is surrounded by the middle layer, the cortex, which consists of long thin cells that give the hair its elasticity and colour. The outer hair layer, known as the cuticle, consists of hundreds of tiny, overlapping scales.

Hair grows from the hair follicle, which is an enclosed sac situated below the surface of the scalp. The follicles, which contain the hair roots, are fed by blood carrying nutrients, hence the importance of good circulation to healthy hair. It is the supply of nutrients which determines the health of the hair as it emerges from the scalp and continues to grow. Hair grows at the rate of about half an inch a month, although this speeds up somewhat during summer, and slows down with age. Once hair leaves the follicle it is in fact technically 'dead', but it grows because of continued tissue formation within the follicle.

Halfway along the hair follicle are located the sebaceous glands which secrete the oil that gives healthy hair its natural sheen. It is a disturbance in the production of sebum by these glands which results in hair that is over dry or greasy. For instance, if the glands become blocked or are underactive, the hair will be dry, whereas if the glands are overactive the result will be hair that is greasy.

Both your natural hair colour, and whether it is straight or curly, are determined by hereditary factors. In those who have curly hair, it is the actual shape of the hair follicle which forces the emerging hair to develop waves. The number of individual hairs you have on your head depends on your natural hair colour, although it will be in the range of 90,000 to 140,000. Blondes have the most hairs since their hair is thinner than that of dark people, and redheads have the least number of hairs, although theirs will often look more abundant since it is generally the thickest. Nothing can alter the number of hair roots or the texture of your hair, apart from the natural changes which occur with age.

FOODS FOR HEALTHY HAIR

As mentioned above, the necessary nutrients must be available if you are to have healthy hair. The advice contained in Chapter 2 applies equally to hair and skin, but there are also certain nutrients of particular importance to hair health. The B complex vitamins, and especially pantothenic acid, influence hair growth, oil production and colour, so an ample supply of these is essential. Vitamins A and C also have a part to play in the production of healthy hair, and vitamin E encourages hair growth by carrying oxygen to the hair roots. To ensure an adequate intake of the essential fatty acids, it is worth including two teaspoons of sunflower or safflower oil in the daily diet. Since the hair is formed from keratin, which is itself a protein-like substance, the diet also needs to include adequate quantities of protein in the form of meat, fish, dairy produce, pulses or nuts. Of the minerals, zinc, copper, iron and iodine are essential to healthy hair. Copper is widely available in food, while liver, kidneys, wholegrains and molasses are good sources of iron. The only foods that contain appreciable quantities of iodine are seafoods.

Your hair, like your skin, is affected not only by diet and health, but also by tension. In a person who is tense the muscles at the base of the neck are constricted, and this impedes the flow of blood to the scalp, resulting in weak hair growth.

WHAT HAIR CARE REALLY MEANS

Another characteristic which hair shares with skin is that it will fall into one of three categories, namely dry, greasy or normal. The care you give your hair will be influenced by its type, but as with skin care there are certain basic guidelines which apply to all types.

A mistake people often make is to wash their hair too frequently, when in fact this is likely to do more harm than good. Shampoos may make hair clean, but at the same time they remove its natural oils and protective acid coating.

A shampoo once or twice a week is enough for most hair, and even very greasy hair should not be washed any more frequently than is absolutely necessary, since this may further stimulate the already overactive sebaceous glands. Some people like to wash their hair every day or every other day because they believe clean hair and scalp equals healthy hair. If you are washing your hair more than twice a week, it is best to use one of the special extra-gentle shampoos designed for frequent use.

You can make your own protein-enriched shampoo which will act as a conditioner and shampoo combined by mixing your usual amount of shampoo in a cup with an egg and 1/3 cup cold water. Beat together well, and use in the normal way.

A dry shampoo is not advisable, since this simply absorbs

the oil on the hair shaft and scalp, rather than removing it. The result is a clogged, dirty scalp, and hair that will need very vigorous brushing to remove its coating of powder. However, if you are desperate, you can use a coarse meal, such as oatmeal or cornmeal, to remove dust and grime in between shampooing.

While on the subject of brushing, the old idea of a hundred brush strokes a day is no longer in favour, since it creates too much friction, and overstimulates the oil glands. However, you should still brush your hair regularly both to free it of dust, dead cells and tangles, and to stimulate the scalp. A brush which has bristles with rounded tips is best, since it is less likely to scratch the scalp or tear and split the hair. A rubber cushioned brush is the easiest to clean, and is more flexible for gentle styling.

These days there are all sorts of different brushes for various purposes. For instance, a semi radial brush (which most hairdressers tend to use) is best for smooth blow drying, and can be used either to straighten or wave the hair, depending on the angle at which you hold it. One with well spaced bristles will achieve the best results.

If your hair is short you are best to use a brush with short, densely spaced bristles. A vent angle brush, which has lots of space between the bristles, is better for getting the tangles out of longer hair, and if used for blow drying helps give extra bounce and lift to the hair. Radial brushes, which have a completely circular base, are the best choice for styling curls while blow drying, and the larger the brush, the larger the curls.

When it comes to combs, there is also a bewildering selection. Wide tooth or afro combs, as the name implies, are designed for very coarse or tightly curled hair, while a fine toothed tail comb, with a slim metal rod at one end, is used for lifting sections of hair while blow drying, roller setting, or for coaxing hair back into shape without upsetting the overall style. If using an ordinary comb, choose a plastic one with rounded teeth, using the larger end initially to ease it through the hair, and the fine end to get a smooth, even finish.

The most effective way to brush the hair is to bend forward from the waist with the head down towards the ground, and brush from the nape of the neck forwards towards the forehead. Short or shoulder-length hair can be brushed right from the roots to the ends in one stroke, but if your hair is long you should use two strokes for the length of each hair, to avoid stretching it.

Make just before or after brushing the time when you treat yourself to a scalp massage. Like brushing, this stimulates the circulation, dislodges dirt and dandruff, and encourages hair growth. To give yourself a massage, spread your fingers fanwise and slip them through the hair. With your thumbs pressed behind your ears, press down on your scalp with your fingertips. Now rotate your fingers so that they move the scalp over the bony structure of the head – you'll feel your skin move and the scalp tingle. Move up an inch at a time until you have covered the whole head. This sounds rather complicated, but in fact it is a very simple procedure, and takes only a few minutes to perform. Massage your scalp daily if you find the time, or at the very least once a week (this is especially important for those suffering from dandruff or falling hair).

THE RIGHT WAY TO WASH YOUR HAIR

There is both a right and a wrong way to wash your hair, and many people use the wrong way, shampooing much too vigorously, applying too much shampoo, and not rinsing it out properly afterwards.

When washing your hair, always use warm, not hot, water, preferably from a shower or hair spray. Once your hair is wet (and not before) apply just a small quantity of shampoo, tipping it on to the palm of your hand and rubbing the hands together. Never apply shampoo directly to the hair since this makes it much more difficult to get an even distribution. Work the shampoo gently but firmly all over your scalp using a circular motion. It is this massaging of the scalp which encourages good circulation, as mentioned above, as well as ensuring that the hair is really clean. Continue to massage the shampoo in for several minutes, using the tips of your fingers rather than the nails.

Only if your hair is really dirty does it need a second application of shampoo, despite what it usually tells you on the bottle. After shampooing give your hair a really good rinse, and go on rinsing it even after you think it is clean, in order to remove every last trace of soap. Hair that is really clean should squeak when rubbed gently between the fingers.

CHOOSING A SHAMPOO

Whatever your hair type, the shampoo you use is of the utmost importance, but choice is made difficult by the bewildering variety of products available. In fact the chemical make-up of all shampoos is virtually the same, since almost all use a chemical detergent as a cleanser. There is a soap-based shampoo on the market but it needs very careful rinsing out with an acid rinse to remove the soap. The difference between the various products lies in the amount of detergent used (a mild shampoo uses less), the quality of the bases, and in the use of any additional ingredients.

The cheaper shampoos usually use petroleum based oils (like washing-up liquid), and they may also include chemical foam boosters and foam stabilizers. Some of the harsher detergents can strip the natural oils from the hair, and may even damage the hair itself, as well as stimulating the sebaceous glands to produce more oil than needed, so that the hair becomes extra greasy. The better quality shampoos, and those found in health food shops, are more likely to be based on vegetable oils, and are unlikely to contain animal ingredients or to have been tested on animals (see page 10).

Many shampoos contain added ingredients, such as herbs which are noted for their beneficial effect on the hair, although there is some doubt about whether their inclusion makes any difference to hair condition since shampoo is left on the hair for such a short time. Particularly common are such hair helpers as nettle, rosemary, chamomile and jojoba. Shampoos on sale in the health food shop often have a higher proportion of such natural ingredients, whereas some of the cheaper shampoos may have added colour and scent to give the desired herbal effect.

Protein or vitamin-enriched shampoos seem to have little effect on the hair, and baby shampoos may not be any milder, since they often just exclude ingredients which may sting the eyes. Most shampoos are mildly alkaline, since this makes them more effective at cleansing the hair, but shampoo which is too alkaline will unbalance the natural acid coating of the hair. When a highly alkaline shampoo is first used it makes the hair look as if it has more body because it swells the hair shaft from within by temporarily increasing its diameter, but this effect is only short term because the interior of the hair is destroyed. A shampoo which is acid (i.e. has a low pH) has the opposite effect, tightening the cuticle scales and shrinking the diameter of the hair. However, an acid shampoo may help the condition of hair that has been coloured or permed, since both these practices leave an alkaline imbalance. Hair that is healthy has a pH of around 5.5 so it is worth looking for a shampoo with about the same pH balance, say between 5 and 8.

CONDITIONING
The time to apply a hair conditioner is after your hair is thoroughly cleansed. These products are especially helpful

for long hair, where the overlapping scales which cover the outer layer of hair often get roughed up as it grows. A conditioner helps to smooth these scales down, and to give shining hair which is easier to comb and manage. Hair that is coloured, permed, or exposed to sun also benefits from a conditioner. In the normal way, dry hair should be conditioned once a week, normal hair once a fortnight, and greasy hair not more than once a month. If your hair is tangly this is a sign that it needs a good conditioner. When applying your conditioner, do not use too much (a dollop about the size of a 10p piece should be sufficient depending on the length of your hair), and be sure to wash it out properly. First lightly towel dry the hair, then apply the conditioner and comb it gently through the hair.

All conditioners are basically a combination of oils or waxes, detergents and emulsifiers, with optional extra ingredients such as herbs or protein. Those on sale in the health food shop have a larger amount of natural ingredients, often incorporating herbal extracts with gentle plant and vegetable oils and essences. They usually exclude animal ingredients too, although most conditioners will contain animal protein.

After conditioning, rinse your hair again, adding cider vinegar or lemon juice to the rinse water to remove all vestiges of soap, and to restore the hair's natural acid coating. Lemon juice is usually used on blonde hair since it acts as a mild bleach.

DRYING AND STYLING

It is important to dry your hair correctly, since it can be easily damaged when wet. First of all wrap your head in a clean towel for a few minutes to remove excess moisture, but refrain from rubbing it with the towel. When your hair is wet always use a comb, since brushing will stretch and tear it. Start with the ends of the hair and work up towards the scalp.

The kindest way to dry your hair is naturally, and finger drying (where the hair is styled by using the fingers) is becoming increasingly popular. If you want to use a hairdryer always have it on the coolest setting, since heat dries out the hair. Most damage is done by over drying, so avoid holding the dryer in one area for too long, and always stop drying a few minutes before your hair feels completely dry. For the same reason, it is advisable not to use attachments like brushes or nozzles, since these concentrate the heat too much, or to hold the dryer any closer than six inches from the head. Heated hair rollers or curling tongs also tend to damage the hair, so keep these for use before special occasions only.

If you want to use rollers, choose sponge ones, or wrap ordinary rollers in several layers of toilet paper or tissues to prevent them tearing the hair. Lemon juice combed through the hair after rinsing acts as a natural setting lotion, or you can add gelatine to the final rinse water.

It goes without saying that your hair will never look good unless it is really well cut. Good hairdressers are hard to find, so if you know one stick with him. Unless you have very definite ideas about the style you want, you are best to put yourself in his hands – a good hairdresser will give you a style that not only takes account of your face shape, but also your height, weight, manner of dress, etc.

THE PERILS OF PERMING

Hair perming is very much in vogue at the moment, and although today's perms are softer than they used to be, they can still wreak considerable damage on the hair. Not surprising, perhaps, when you consider that a perm is bombarding the hair with powerful and disruptive chemicals that actually realign the cellular structure of the hair. The chemicals may also affect the scalp, giving rise to irritation or inflammation, especially in women with sensitive skins.

If you still feel you would like to go ahead, do ensure that your perm is given by a reputable hairdresser, and opt for one of the softer, body perms.

SOME NATURAL HAIR CARE PRODUCTS

If you suffer from dry hair, a conditioner used after shampooing will, as already mentioned, put some life and lustre back into your hair. An occasional oil treatment also helps improve dry hair. To use this, apply a warmed vegetable oil to your hair, massage it well in, and wrap your head in a towel which has been wrung out in hot water. Leave this on for at least quarter of an hour before shampooing. Cider vinegar or lemon juice in the final rinse water will help to remove any last traces of oil.

An egg yolk shampoo is a gentle cleanser which is especially suited to dry hair. Simply mix one or two egg yolks (depending on the length of your hair) with a little warm water. Make sure the water is not too hot when you add it, or you'll end up with scrambled egg! Apply this mixture to your hair, wrap your head in a towel, and leave for several minutes before rinsing thoroughly. There is no need to apply any other shampoo.

Eggs can also be used as the basis of a protein treatment, which helps restore condition to any hair type. Beat together two eggs, one tablespoonful vegetable oil, one tablespoonful of glycerine and one teaspoonful of cider vinegar. Apply after shampooing and rinsing, and leave on for fifteen minutes. Rinse well. You will find other suggestions for natural hair care products you can prepare yourself included in Chapter 11.

A CHANGE OF COLOUR

An estimated 40 per cent of women will at some time succumb to the temptation to change the natural shade of their hair, despite the fact that some of the chemicals used have been proved to be carcinogenic (i.e. cancer inducing) in animals. Research on this still continues, although it is currently hampered by lack of funds.

It was in the 1970s that hair dyes were first suspected, when research conducted in both America and Britain independently reached the same conclusion, namely that some of the ingredients used in hair dyes are carcinogenic in large doses in animals. There is still no proof of their effect on humans, although it is known that substances are easily absorbed through the scalp and into the blood-stream.

Testing is complicated by the fact that different products vary in their ingredients and their proportions, which means ideally that all the individual ingredients need to be tested in varying strengths.

Permanent dyes penetrate the hair's cortex layer with the aid of hydrogen peroxide, destroy the keratin structure and create porosity. These dyes will gradually eat away and destroy the delicate structure of the hair, as will the use of semi-permanent dyes. Colour rinses, which are used like a shampoo but in order to highlight the hair's natural shade are much safer, although they are not natural.

If you are planning to use any of these colourants it is essential to do an allergy test first, and instructions to this effect should appear on the product.

Alternatives in the natural field are limited, and are likely to produce a less dramatic effect, but they are safe. Most need to be used repeatedly over a period of time before there is any marked difference in hair colour. Test any hair dye on the ends of your hair before applying it to your head (the ends are more porous than the rest of the hair, and enable you to see the results before it is too late).

Herbs have been used for many centuries as colouring agents, the most common being sage for dark or greying hair, and chamomile for fair hair. To use herbs as colourants, make them into a rinse and apply after shampooing. For instance, to lighten brown hair, add 2–4 tablespoonsful of chamomile flowers to a pint (550ml) of boiling water and leave it to stand for up to three hours. Strain, and use the resulting liquid to rinse the hair several times, holding a basin under your head to catch the liquid so that you can re-use it.

An alternative which is more effective, although also more trouble, is to make your own herbal hair dye. This is produced by taking four tablespoonsful of the herb of your choice and leaving them to stand in a cupful of boiling water for at least twenty minutes. Strain and mix the liquid to a paste with kaolin (a fine clay powder available from chemists). Apply this mixture to the roots of your hair, and them comb it through. Leave on for between twenty minutes and one hour, depending on the desired effect – the longer you leave it, the more marked will be the change.

Rhubarb root is the strongest of all the herbal lighteners, and can be used to brighten and lift the colour of all hair types. It will give gold highlights even on the first application. Boil 2 oz. of the root in two pints of water, cover and simmer for an hour. Cool and strain and use repeatedly as a rinse, as with the chamomile described above. For best results let the hair dry naturally in the sunlight.

One effective natural hair colourant which can be purchased ready-made is henna. This imparts a reddish tinge to dark hair, without changing the chemical structure of the hair as other dyes do. Instead it coats the hair and gives it extra body – in fact, henna is often used as a hair conditioner. Henna preparations are now widely available, but the best to choose is the all-natural henna, since the compound henna may have added synthetic ingredients.

Henna is also available now in combination with other natural colouring agents, such as chamomile, rhubarb root or walnut, so that colours other than the characteristic reddish shade may be obtained. Henna comes in various forms, such as the traditional powder, or in a cream, which is as easy to use as shampoo, but whichever you choose do make sure that you follow the instructions carefully or you may find the results rather unpredictable!

YOUR HAIR CARE CHART

Hair Type	How to Recognize It	Shampooing	Special Care
Normal	Shiny without being greasy. Fairly easy to manage. Looks good for about a week after shampooing.	Wash once a week following general instructions. Use a conditioner every other week.	Massage daily. Use a protein conditioner twice a month.
Greasy	Looks good for a day or two but quickly becomes lank.	Wash as little as possible, at the most twice a week. Pay particular attention to massaging shampoo in. Rinse thoroughly adding cider vinegar or lemon juice to rinse water.	Massage daily. Use a dry shampoo like bran or oatmeal. Use a protein conditioner once a month.
Dry	Difficult to control. Looks dull with dry ends. Scalp often feels itchy.	Wash once a week using a cream shampoo. Use a conditioner each time.	Massage daily. Use an oil treatment once a fortnight.

CHAPTER SEVEN

A PAIR OF SPARKLING EYES

It takes only a poor night's sleep, a bout of crying, or a heavy cold to make your eyes look dull, red and strained – hardly conducive to beauty, you must admit. Clear white sparkling eyes are an essential part of looking beautiful, but the eyes are even more directly affected by external factors than the skin and hair.

VITAMINS
The first requisite for beautiful eyes is a good diet which supplies plenty of vitamin A. This vitamin is closely connected with good eyesight and clear eyes, and especially with the ability to see in dim light or the dark. Foods rich in vitamin A include butter and margarine, oily fish, and orange and yellow fruits and vegetables. Other vitamins essential to good eyesight are vitamins B2, C and D. Where there is a lack of vitamin B2, eyes often become bloodshot, itchy and watery.

Vitamin A is especially important to those who use their eyes a lot (e.g. reading, typing, etc.), since these people use up extra vitamin A. Equally important is to see that you work in plenty of light, which should come from above, behind or the side, but not from the front since this tends to make you squint, thus encouraging wrinkles as well as poor eyesight.

If you use your eyes a lot, try to rest them at intervals during the day. This can be done by palming, which simply means covering both eyes with the palms of your hands so that all light is excluded. Keep your eyes covered, but open, for five minutes.

EYE EXERCISES

Eye exercises are quick and easy to do and are worth the effort since they help the eyesight by strengthening the muscles, while at the same time reducing eye strain. A good exercise is to roll your eyes round in circles while keeping your head still. Rotate the eyes in each direction, trying to do this twelve times a day. Another simple but effective exercise is to hold your index finger about three inches from your face. Look at it closely, and then quickly extend your arm as far as it will go in front of you, all the time following your finger with your eyes. Then bring your finger back to within a few inches of your face. Repeat this several times.

HELP FOR RED, PUFFY EYES

Refresh tired, reddened eyes by placing a slice of cucumber over the closed lids while you rest with your feet up. You'll find this very cooling and refreshing. Tea bags, too, can be used for the same purpose – but wring them out first!

Bathe tired, strained eyes with an eye bath made from the herb eyebright, used for centuries for this purpose and still included in many of today's commercial eyewashes. Prepare the lotion by pouring a cupful of boiling water over one teaspoon of the dried herb and leave until cool. Strain and use the liquid to bathe the eyes. Witchhazel can be used in the same way, or try half a teaspoonful of salt dissolved in a glass of mineral water. These methods are much kinder to the eyes than commercial eye drops which clear the eyes by forcing dilated blood vessels to contract.

A gentle massage can also help relieve tired, aching eyes. Using the tips of the middle fingers, exert gentle pressure starting from the bridge of the nose and tapping across the eyelids and back under the eyes half a dozen times. Then press quite hard on either side of the bridge of the nose close to the inner eye.

Dark circles and swelling under the eyes can be caused by lack of sleep, which is another good reason for getting plenty of it. Eight hours a night is the ideal amount for most people, so when you are out late, try and make up for those lost hours the following night. Reduce swelling or bags under the eyes by applying ice-cold witchhazel, water or milk. Dab this on with cotton wool.

Puffiness around the eyes can also be caused by applying the wrong sort of cosmetics. The skin around the eyes is very thin and delicate, containing no sebaceous glands and with little circulation. This means it needs extra care. Never use astringents, heavy creams, or face masks around the eyes, since these will stretch the skin, leading to puffiness and premature wrinkles.

Many women find that they become allergic to a particular brand of eye make up, even after using it for a number of years. If you develop sore red eyes all of a sudden, stop using any make up for a few days and see if the condition clears up. If it does, then it is worth trying another cosmetic brand, such as one of the hypo-allergenic ranges which are produced for those with sensitive skin. If the condition persists even without the use of make up, you should see your doctor without delay.

USING A MOISTURIZER

Regular moisturizing is as important for the eye area as it is for the rest of the face, since it helps to soften and lubricate the skin and to delay the formation of wrinkles. However, you need to choose your moisturizer with care, opting for a special eye cream which is very light in texture. Many people have found that an eye cream is more effective if it contains vitamin E – buy a product containing this, or add the contents of a capsule to your eye cream. There's a recipe for vitamin E eye cream on page 132.

A light vegetable oil such as almond or avocado is also ideal for the eye area, but whatever you choose, never apply too much cream or oil around the eyes as this can cause puffiness due to retention of fluid.

Unless you apply your eye cream correctly you will be doing your eyes more harm than good. Here's the right way to apply cream to the eye area: using the pad of your forefinger, start at the inner corner of the eye and very gently spread the cream over the eyelid to the outer corner, then back under the eye to the centre. You should also use this method when applying any kind of eye make up, and when removing it too.

REMOVING EYE MAKE UP
As far as this is concerned, always use a remover designed specifically for the eyes. While other lotions may effectively remove the make up, many will also make the eyes red and sore. Make it a habit to remove eye make up every night without fail. It may be the last thing you feel like doing when you are tired, but it is worth the effort or your neglect will show in spots, and sparse, weakened eyelashes.

When removing eye make up, rub the cotton wool or remover pad gently down over the eyelid and upper lashes, then open the eyes and wipe the lower lashes, working towards the inner corner of the eye as described above. Make sure you remove all traces of the remover, since most of these tend to be greasy, and could cause whiteheads if left on the skin.

PLUCKING THE EYEBROWS
This should be done without altering the basic shape, and for this reason you should only remove hairs from below the eyebrows and from each end. When correctly shaped, the brows should start above the inner corner of the eye, with the highest part of the curve above the outer rim of the iris, and ending at the point where a diagonal line drawn from the nose to the outer corner of the eye would cross the brow. (See Fig. 3).

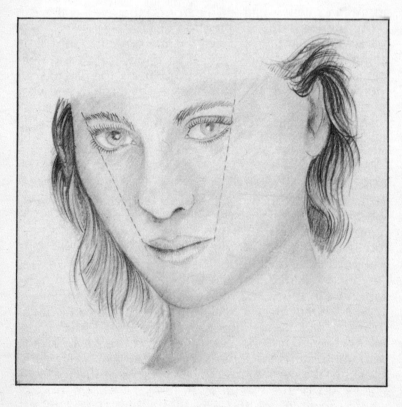

Figure 3

The best time for plucking the eyebrows is after a bath, while your skin is still warm, to minimize any redness or soreness. Always pull the hairs out in the direction in which they grow. Finish up by dabbing a little mild toner on to the plucked area to discourage any redness.

CHAPTER EIGHT

LOOKING AFTER YOUR TEETH

Did you know that 37 per cent of adults in the U.K. over the age of sixteen have none of their own teeth? It is a staggering statistic, and unless you take proper care of your teeth, you could be well on the way to acquiring a set of dentures yourself. Yet research conducted during the past 30 years has shown that both dental decay, and the gum disease which so often accompanies it, are almost completely preventable.

The dental profession is in fact gradually becoming more concerned with prevention, and more aware of the role of nutrition and general health in relation to tooth decay. This is reflected in the recent formation of the British Dental Society for Clinical Nutrition, a body which plans to investigate and collate research on the importance of nutrition to the way a dentist works. This society is open to all qualified dental practitioners, with associate membership offered to dental hygienists, therapists and students in their final two years of training.

It is a move that is long overdue, although during the last 15 years the rate of decay has begun to fall, due firstly to a reduction in sugar consumption (down 20 per cent in the last ten years), and to more widespread use of fluoride toothpaste, leading to less decay in children's teeth.

HOW TO CLEAN YOUR TEETH
Ideally teeth should be cleaned after every meal, but one thorough cleaning each day will do far more good than any number of hurried brushings. A quick brushing is a waste of time because although your teeth may appear clean,

they will still be coated with an invisible layer of plaque, and it is the presence of this sticky, transparent substance which leads to decay. In fact, even with a normal brushing you can still miss as much as 80 per cent of the plaque.

Night time is the time for really thorough cleansing, when you should devote at least three minutes to brushing your teeth. If you are unsure whether or not you are getting your teeth really clean, invest occasionally in a packet of disclosing tablets. These contain a food dye (which you are not expected to swallow!), to colour any remaining dirt or plaque bright red so that there is no mistaking where you have omitted to clean.

It is important not only to choose the right toothbrush, but also to renew it regularly – about every three or four months, or as soon as the tufts begin to splay out. Most dentists recommend a nylon brush in preference to a natural one, and advise using a flat tufted brush with a small head, since this makes it easier to reach the awkward areas. They also recommend a medium to soft brush, since one that is too hard tends to wear away the enamel and push back the gums from the tooth margin.

There are a number of theories on how best to clean your teeth, but the consensus of dental opinion seems to back using a circular motion with the brush, ensuring that all surfaces are cleaned. Do not be afraid to touch the gums with the brush, since they benefit from gentle stimulation to improve the circulation.

Using dental floss may seem like an awful performance at first, but it is really quite simple once you get used to it, and it does remove any hidden particles of food from between the teeth, and from underneath the flap of skin where the gums meet the teeth. Waxed floss is easier to use if you have fillings, although the unwaxed variety is easier for getting around the teeth. For those unfamiliar with floss, it is a length of fine nylon thread, which is wound round the forefingers of each hand thus giving a taut thread for sliding up and down between the teeth to the gum margin.

Toothpaste is not in fact essential for the removal of plaque, although most people prefer to use it, and it does help to keep the mouth fresh. Fluoride, which is added to an increasing number of pastes (see next page) helps to strengthen the outer enamel and thus render it less susceptible to decay, but it has no effect on gum disease, which affects 99 per cent of those with their own teeth and is the main reason for adults losing their teeth.

Most of the toothpastes on the market are made to a similar basic formula. This consists of an abrasive (30–50 per cent), which is usually a mineral material such as chalk, alumina or synthetic variations, and is used to help clean and polish the teeth. A humectant (usually glycerine derived from animals) is included to produce the right consistency paste, and a detergent is added to give foaming properties. Flavourings and colourings are usually synthetic (and may even contain sweetening!), and in the case of toothpastes specifically for sensitive teeth, there will also be some anaesthetizing agents. Preservatives may be included to make sure the sugar does not react with other ingredients to cause fermentation, and various cosmetic ingredients (such as synthetic plasticizers and aerators) ensure that the toothpaste behaves correctly.

There are a number of toothpastes available in the health food shop, although these vary widely. Some follow the basic formula described above but with added plant extracts; while others contain less or no abrasive, no detergent, no or fewer synthetics, and pure flavourings. Bases are usually natural, and glycerine, where used, is from non-animal sources. Various claims are made for such pastes, for instance that they are not tested on animals, contain no sugar, sweetener, preservatives or chemicals etc. Texture and taste vary considerably, so it is worth trying several brands until you find one to your liking.

FOR AND AGAINST FLUORIDE

Fluoride, as mentioned before, is added to an increasing number of toothpastes, and the dental profession mostly backs this move since it believes that this substance is effective in helping to fight tooth decay.

Fluoride can be administered in various ways: in toothpaste, by the dentist, in drops, tablets or via the water supply, and it is the latter which causes the most controversy. The strong pro-fluoridation lobby (including most dentists) claims that this is the most effective way of reducing decay (by 50 to 60 per cent), while opponents say that it is undemocratic to apply compulsory medication in this way, and that it has side effects, including an increased risk of cancer. Certainly too much fluoride can cause mottling of the teeth, an uneven discolouration which is difficult to remove. There is concern that fluoridation may adversely affect children who are poorly nourished, such as those who are low in magnesium (a common deficiency). Claims have also been made for an apparent link between fluoride and cot deaths, genetic damage, birth defects and allergies.

Particular concern centres around bottle fed babies, who ingest high rates of fluoride because of their high intake of fluid in relation to body weight, and this could give them as much as 150 times more fluoride than a breastfed baby. The Food and Drug Administration in America concluded that fluoride could cause possible harm to the foetus if taken during pregnancy, and that it had no benefit to the teeth of the mother or baby. Fluoridation has also been linked with kidney failure in children. In Victoria, Australia, for instance, there has been a 63 per cent increase in renal failure since fluoridated water was introduced in 1977.

Holland banned fluoride in 1976 on the grounds of health hazards, as did Chile in 1973 after 23 years of trials, mainly because of the harmful effects on children. In

Sweden also it was banned in 1971 because of concern that it may be harmful to the unborn and the very young.

In this country at the moment some five million people have fluoridated water, and this usually dates back to before 1973 when the Water Act was introduced. If the Water Bill becomes law, the onus will be on each water authority to choose whether or not to fluoridate, but at the moment most seem to be against the move. In any case, there are tremendous problems to be overcome first, for all the health authorities in an area covered by a water authority would have to be in agreement, the cost of equipment would be substantial, and the question of liability in cases of·fluoride causing illness would have to be sorted out. If you are unsure whether your water is fluoridated, contact your local water authority.

In the meantime, there is concern over children swallowing fluoride toothpastes, especially in areas where the water is fluoridated, for tests have shown that this could result in a daily intake of three times higher than the safety level of 1 mg. Even the pro-fluoridation British Dental Health Foundation admits that fluoride pastes should not be swallowed in large quantities because of their toxicity. There have been widespread reports of apparent side effects from using such toothpastes, for instance cases of mouth ulcers, stomach and bowel disorders.

WHAT IS TOOTH DECAY?

Tooth decay starts when bacteria in the mouth set to work on food particles. The bacteria need food to provide energy for breeding, and they break down food into the sticky film known as plaque. This protects them from cleaning, attracts more food debris, and provides their ideal, oxygen-free environment for breeding. As the bacteria break down the food into the sugar they need for energy, a by-product called lactic acid is formed, and it is this which attacks the tooth enamel.

At this stage you will be unaware of the decay. It is only when it starts to penetrate the softer dentine inside the tooth that you may become aware of unusual sensitivity when eating hot, cold or sweet foods. Toothache begins when the decay reaches the central nerve of the tooth.

The accumulation of plaque can also lead to gum inflammation and bleeding (known as gingivitis), which are early warning signs of gum disease. In this case the plaque collects at the gum margins, especially under the flap of skin around the edges of the teeth.

Just as important as regular and thorough brushing of your teeth, is to make frequent visits to your dentist. Most people have a dread of the dentist, imagining that they will be subjected to all sorts of excruciating torture, but with the modern methods of today, dental treatment is rarely painful. You certainly should not put off going to the dentist, and should make it a habit to visit him every six months for a check up. A dentist will also be able to give you any advice you may need on cosmetic problems, such as crooked or chipped teeth.

For the past 150 years, a dental amalgam has been used for filling teeth, this being an alloy of silver and mercury mixed with other metals such as nickel and copper so it can withstand the tremendous crushing and grinding forces generated by our back teeth. However, there is increasing concern over the inclusion of mercury, which it is believed can lead to poisoning of the individual over a prolonged period, due to gradual leaching of the mercury into the system. As far back as 1845 the American Society of Dental Practitioners was so concerned that it declared the use of amalgam as a form of malpractice, and this caused a major split within the dental profession. Debate centres on whether or not mercury escapes from the filling, but the evidence seems conclusive. The mercury content of a new amalgam filling is 50 per cent, falling to a level of around 28 per cent after a few years.

Mercury from fillings may be absorbed into the system in several ways. Small particles break away from the filling and are swallowed, being converted in the digestive tract by anaerobic bacteria into methyl-mercury which is then absorbed. Mercury vapour discharged from the fillings is inhaled and enters the blood stream via the lungs. And the need to replace fillings about every five years aggravates the situation when the old filling is drilled out and replaced with a new more toxic one. The dentist and his assistants, who are constantly exposed to mercury, may be at greater risk, a situation which is currently being carefully monitored in America.

Low level mercury toxicity can produce a wide range of symptoms, such as headaches, general fatigue, gastro-intestinal problems, walking difficulties, joint and muscle problems, asthma, skin complaints, and disorders of the central nervous system.

Modern composite materials have replaced amalgam to a certain extent, but are so far only suitable for the front teeth where they are not subjected to the same pressure. These are a mixture of organic resin, which is a kind of plastic, with inorganic fillers and a coupling agent. They also have the advantage of being colour-matched to an individual's own teeth.

Trials are currently being conducted by the National Health Service with a new material called occlusin, which appears to have the necessary strength. It is stronger than other composites because it contains more powdered glass and less resin, with a fast acting bonding agent. It has already undergone extensive tests, and is available privately from a limited number of British dentists. Another new dental technique called fissure sealing applies a plastic coating on the tooth surface to stop invading food organisms attaching themselves and damaging the tooth.

Bad breath is as unpleasant and embarrassing for the sufferer as it is for those he comes into contact with. If your digestion is functioning efficiently you are unlikely to suffer from bad breath – unless, of course, you have just indulged in a highly seasoned meal or a portion of garlic bread! Freshen your breath naturally by chewing fresh parsley or watercress, or by using rosewater or lavender water as a mouth wash. Commercial antiseptic mouth-washes are very strong, and can upset the natural balance of your mouth, but you can easily make your own by mixing equal parts of rosewater and water.

DIET AND YOUR TEETH

Diet has a large part to play in dental health, and it has been proved that plaque builds up most in those who eat a lot of refined carbohydrates and sugar. It is therefore important to try and restrict your sugar intake, and to make sure that your diet includes plenty of crisp, crunchy foods like raw vegetables and wholemeal bread. Wholefoods are good for the teeth since the hard fibre helps firm the gums and clean the teeth, whereas fibreless refined foods allow particles to accumulate on the teeth in a sticky mass, and bind sugary substances where they can do most harm. The gums need this friction to keep them hard, and the wholefoods also help remove plaque and have earned themselves the names of 'detergent foods' with some dentists.

However, wholefoods only benefit the teeth if they are free from sugar. As Surgeon-Captain Cleave, who wrote *The Saccharine Disease* (Weight, 1974) says, 'It is perfectly true that refined carbohydrates are a prime cause (of dental decay), but it does not necessarily follow that unrefined carbohydrates can not be a cause. If they take the form of stale, coarse wholemeal bread, and hard fruits and vegetables, no peridontal disease will follow their consumption.'

The fact that sugar consumption is inextricably linked with tooth decay was clearly demonstrated during World

War II, when dental surveys showed that during sugar rationing decay fell dramatically, only to increase again when sugar once more became widely available.

Similar evidence was produced by a unique three year nutrition project recently carried out at Ashley Down in Bristol, during which time both parents and children were encouraged to reduce their intake of sugar and sweet foods, and to increase their intake of fibre. A dental check up at an infant school towards the end of the three year period revealed a ten per cent reduction in the number of children needing dental care.

It is not only what you eat but when that is important when trying to prevent tooth decay. Frequent small snacks spell disaster, since they produce an acid medium in which the bacteria thrive. That is why the number of times you eat sugar is one of the most important factors in determining the rate of decay. For this reason it is better to eat sweets (if you must) at the end of a meal rather than between meals.

Research has shown that cheese is an excellent food to help clean the teeth, whereas (contrary to popular belief) apples are good for firming the gums but have little effect on the teeth. This is because they contain acids which have no beneficial effect on the acid in the mouth, and that is the crucial factor in decay.

The answer therefore seems to be to eat as many wholefoods and as little sugar as possible – a diet which will benefit your health as well as your teeth. A baby's teeth are formed before birth, which is why it is so important for a woman's diet to contain sufficient calcium during pregnancy. When your children begin to teethe, chewing on a stale bread crust, or a stick of raw carrot will ease any tenderness and irritation. Once your child starts eating solid foods, do your best not to encourage a sweet tooth, by keeping sugar to an absolute minimum and using it only when necessary (e.g. in a very tart fruit dish). Sweetened drinks like fruit squashes and fizzy drinks should be replaced with fresh fruit juices, which can be served diluted with water to make them go further. If your child is used to drinking fresh juice right from the start, then the squash will seem far too sweet to him.

Children should be discouraged right from the start from eating too many sweets, hard though this is when they are bombarded with advertising, with eye level displays at supermarket check-outs, and with friends who seem to have unlimited access to packets of sweets. Offer your child fresh fruit, raw celery or carrot, or nuts as alternatives. Obviously it is impossible to prevent children from eating sweets altogether, especially once they start going to parties and to friends' houses, but it helps if you explain to them the reasons why sweet eating is bad (i.e. for teeth and health), and the importance of brushing their teeth afterwards. As mentioned above, the best time for eating sweets is at the end of a meal, when the teeth can be cleaned straight away afterwards.

There is a temptation to think that a child's first teeth do not matter, since they are going to fall out naturally, but the permanent teeth are forming underneath the first ones, and even at this early stage they can be irreparably damaged. Dental care should begin as early in life as possible, and almost as soon as a child acquires his first teeth he should have them brushed regularly. He will not understand what it is all about, but it will get him into the habit.

The nutrients your diet needs to contain for strong healthy teeth are the minerals phosphorous and calcium, vitamins A and D, and protein. Vitamin C is essential for healthy gums, and bleeding in this area is often one of the first signs of a vitamin C deficiency.

If you are in the habit of drinking strong tea or coffee, or of smoking cigarettes, your teeth are likely to become yellow and discoloured. Since these practices are bad for your health too, it's worth trying to give them up. However, if all else fails, scrubbing the teeth with lemon peel helps to remove any stains. It is important to rinse your mouth out well after using this, otherwise you create an unnaturally acid medium. A powder for stain removal can be made by mixing three tablespoonsful of bicarbonate of soda and two tablespoonsful of salt. Rub the teeth well with this mixture.

CHAPTER NINE

CARING FOR YOUR HANDS AND FEET

Your hands have a hard life. Not only are they exposed to all kinds of weather conditions, but they are constantly being immersed in water which contains such powerful chemical solutions as washing powder, bleach, washing up liquid, etc. It is little wonder, therefore, that your hands are one of the first parts of the body to show signs of neglect and ageing.

However careful you may be to keep them hidden from view, people tend to notice the state of your hands. That is one good reason for taking care of them; another is that, as with most things, preventing trouble is considerably easier than curing it.

WEAR GLOVES
Rule number one is to protect your hands in such a way that they do not come into direct contact with a constant barrage of chemicals. This means wearing a pair of rubber gloves for all household chores like washing, washing up, and cleaning. They may make you feel ham-fisted, but if you choose a pair of fine rubber gloves you will find that you soon get used to wearing them. And for jobs where your hands will not be immersed in water, cotton gloves can be worn. Keep a pair of rubber gloves in a prominent place next to the sink so that you have no excuse for forgetting to wear them.

MOISTURE
Equally important to the state of your hands is plenty of moisture. However religiously you may wear your gloves, your hands are still going to be immersed in water

frequently (e.g. when bathing or washing yourself), and this tends to dry out the natural oils. The way to counteract this is to apply a nourishing cream every time your hands have been in water, or after every rough job. Once again, a jar or bottle of handcream strategically placed in the kitchen and bathroom will act as a constant reminder. A nourishing lotion you can easily make yourself is half a cup of glycerine mixed with a cup of rosewater. Variations to this basic recipe can be made by adding two tablespoonsful of lemon juice, or by heating two tablespoonsful of glycerine, and adding two tablespoonsful of cornflour and a cupful of rosewater. Other handcream recipes for you to make at home can be found in Chapter 11.

Your hands will also benefit if you replace over-alkaline soaps with glycerine or vegetable-based ones which are less drying. Rinsing your hands in cider vinegar after washing helps to restore the skin's natural acid coating. Always ensure that you dry your hands thoroughly after washing.

If you suffer from poor circulation (suggested by constantly cold hands with a blotchy bluish tinge) always wear warm gloves when you go out in winter, and carefully massage your hands with long stroking movements whenever you apply hand cream. Typing, playing the piano, or exercises like strumming the fingers on a table all help improve circulation. Chilblains benefit from the same treatment, but also ensure that your diet contains ample calcium.

TREATING NEGLECTED HANDS
If your hands have been neglected long enough to get into a very poor state, start by using a well-soaped pumice stone to rub off any roughened skin. Then soak your hands in a mixture of equal parts of salt, Epsom salts and water softener, dissolved in warm water. If you let your hands soak in this mixture for a few minutes you will open the

pores and stimulate the circulation, after which you can rub in a rich hand cream. Repeat this soaking and moisturizing procedure every day until your hands get back to their normal shape.

Treat your hands once or twice a week to a massage with a really rich cream. Once a week precede this by soaking your hands in warmed oil (preferably olive or almond) for between five and thirty minutes. This is a great treatment for dry hands and nails.

Whenever you are using a lemon in the kitchen, keep the skin and pulp and rub this over your hands to whiten and soften them, and to clean your nails and cuticles.

CARE FOR FINGER NAILS

Nails are formed by very tightly packed layers of skin cells which grow from the dermis skin layer. Only half the nail is visible, the other half (known as the matrix) is also oval in shape and extends to the first finger joint. Nails take anything from three to five months to grow, the rate depending upon how healthy you are and your rate of metabolism. Like the hair, nails grow fastest during the summer, and they are also faster growing on whichever hand you use most.

Nails are composed of keratin (as is the hair) which is formed mainly from protein and calcium. That is why a diet rich in these two nutrients is an essential part of healthy nails. Other important nutrients are zinc, potassium and iron, as well as vitamins A and B. Nails that are in poor condition (e.g. with ridges, white spots or flaking) are a sure indication that your general health is below par.

The finger nails, like the hands, have to pay the price for being constantly subjected to abuse, so any hand care programme should incorporate the nails. They will benefit from regular applications of any rich moisturizer, such as a night cream.

Give your nails a regular manicure once a week. First of

all remove any old varnish, if worn, and then shape the nails, using an emery board which is less harsh than a metal file. File in one direction only, from the sides to the centre, since a sawing motion will cause flaking. Nails should be filed round, rather than pointed, although if your nails are short and inclined to break, filing them square helps them to grow evenly. Only use scissors or nail clippers if your nails are badly out of shape or broken.

Clean under the nails with an orange stick tipped with cotton wool. An orange stick should also be used to gently shape the cuticles, to avoid breaking or tearing the skin. The best time to shape the cuticles is after your hands have been in water (for instance after a bath) since this helps to soften the skin ready for shaping. Otherwise, you can soak your fingers in a little vegetable oil, or in warm water and herbal shampoo, for a few minutes during your weekly manicure.

After gently coaxing the cuticles back (avoiding the temptation to cut them), apply a good coating of moisturizer or cuticle cream. You can make your own by mixing two tablespoonsful of petroleum jelly with half a teaspoonful of glycerine. Massage this in well, and then blot away any excess with a tissue.

Buffing the nails helps to improve the circulation, since it stimulates the flow of blood around the nails. Buffing is done with a specially designed pad covered in leather (available from most chemists). When using this, pass the buffer across the whole nail from side to side.

Nail varnishes are very drying, the worst offenders being the pearlized ones (which contain fish scales). For this reason, it is best to go without varnish as often as possible. Varnishes are mainly composed of nitro-cellulose lacquer with pigments and solvents that evaporate, leaving the coloured lacquer to harden on the nails. Plasticizers, colourings, thinning agents and solvents are also added, with the result that the final product may contain as many as 20 different ingredients. Health food shop varnishes have slightly different formulations, leaving out the really harsh chemicals and in some cases adding extra vitamins, minerals and natural oils. These gentler varnishes may not last as long.

When applying varnish, first put on a base coat up the nail from the base to the tip, using as few strokes as possible. Apply at least two coats, leaving time for each to harden, and remembering that although the varnish will quickly feel dry to the touch, it will not harden properly for several hours.

Always remove nail polish at least once a week, since an accumulation of several coats of polish can make nails even more dry and flaky. Nail varnish remover is usually a mixture of acetone (a simple chemical solvent) with water, artificial perfumes and colours. Oil based removers are still based on acetone, but have added oils to improve the condition of the nail and make the remover less drying. You can also counteract this drying by adding a teaspoonful of glycerine to a bottle of acetone. This has the advantage of being considerably cheaper than proprietary brands of remover.

Drinking cider vinegar each day is said to help strengthen nails, as well as being good for your general health. Take a tablespoonful of the vinegar in a glass of water three times a day before meals.

For advice on treating some of the common problems with nails, please turn to page 54.

DON'T FORGET YOUR FEET
With feet, it is often a case of out of sight, out of mind. Because they are hidden away for much of the time, it is easy to forget about looking after them. But feet need regular care not only to make them look good, but to avoid such crippling conditions as corns and callouses, which can turn even a quick trip round the shops into a painful feat(!) of endurance. If conditions like this develop, it is a good

idea to consult a chiropodist.

Ill-fitting shoes are the most likely cause of foot problems, so always choose shoes for comfort rather than fashion. Shoes should support the arch of the foot well, and should allow ample room for the toes.

Keep your feet in good shape with a few simple exercises. First thing in the morning, arch your ankles, bend your toes and flex the whole foot. Walking is one of the best beauty treatments (provided your shoes fit well), while standing on tiptoe is a good exercise and can be practised at odd moments throughout the day.

For feet that are sore and swollen after a long day, relax with your feet higher than your head, and gently massage your legs and feet. Soak your feet in cold water and cider vinegar, in salt water, or in warm water containing a handful of nettle leaves. Cold feet respond well to a massage with olive oil, while an old remedy for tired feet is alternate soaking in hot and cold water, ending with the cold.

Once a week at bathtime give your feet a good going over. While your skin is still warm from the bath rub off any hard skin with a pumice stone. Then trim the nails, cutting and filing as necessary, but following the general advice given for finger nails. Unlike the finger nails, toe nails should be shaped straight across. If rounded or pointed they can cause discomfort or give rise to ingrowing nails. After shaping, massage in a cuticle cream and shape the cuticles with an orange stick.

Clean well around the nails with an orange stick tipped with cotton wool, paying particular attention to the sides of the nails where dirt tends to collect. After this pedicure, rub plenty of moisturizing body lotion all over your feet.

To keep your feet smelling fresh, especially in hot weather, apply a deodorizing talcum powder each morning after washing. Always wash socks or tights daily or, better still, go without if the weather permits.

CHAPTER TEN

HOW TO HAVE A BEAUTIFUL HOLIDAY

As you pack your holiday suitcase, beauty is probably far from your thoughts. After all, the last thing you want to be bothered with while you are away is routine of any sort, including a beauty routine. All the same it is worth sparing a thought before you leave home for a few items which will help you keep up a good appearance while you're away – there is no point in undoing all that good work you've been doing at home!

You may enjoy soaking up the sun, and a deep golden suntan can certainly do wonders for your looks and your morale, but you do need to proceed with caution. Careful sunbathing is beneficial, since it stimulates the whole metabolism as well as the circulation and cell growth; it can relieve asthma, arthritis and acne; and it activates vitamin D production and assists calcium absorption.

Too much sun, on the other hand, is detrimental to your skin, and possibly to your health too. Degenerative changes can take place at the skin's deeper layers, causing premature ageing, with loss of elasticity and the appearance of wrinkles. At the same time, the body may become deficient in vitamin B, and prolonged exposure to the sun (especially by those who do not normally come from a sunny climate) is linked with skin cancer. An increasing number of skin cancer cases are being seen every year, with as many as a quarter of all cancers being those affecting the skin.

A further word of warning to anybody who is taking the contraceptive pill, tranquillizers, antibiotics or antihista-mines. These drugs can cause unusual sun sensitivity, producing a reaction similar to that of an allergy, with sudden violent burning, and inflammation. In such cases, a product offering total sun screening is essential.

You will probably know from bitter experience just how much or how little sun your body can take. The colour of your hair and skin is a good indication, those with a dark complexion being able to tolerate much more sun than the fair-skinned. How easily you tan is determined by a pigment called melanin – dark-skinned people have a lot of it, fair haired people have less, and red heads have virtually none.

According to dermatologists, the majority of white people (78 per cent) have skin of average sensitivity to the sun, i.e. they tan but can burn. Twelve per cent have a very sensitive skin which rarely tans but burns, while eight per cent have what is described as less sensitivity, and these lucky few can tan easily without burning. Only two per cent have an ultra-sensitive skin which never tans and which burns easily.

It is the ultra-violet rays of the sun which give us a tan, and which can burn. The UVB (or short wave) rays are the ones primarily responsible for both tanning and burning. These rays are mostly absorbed by the epidermis (the outer layer of skin), but about ten per cent penetrate to the next skin layer, the dermis. The UVA (or long wave) rays penetrate more deeply, and although they are beneficial in that they help in the synthesis of vitamin D, they are also believed to cause degenerative changes deep within the skin tissue, as mentioned above.

When the skin is exposed to the sun, it has two methods of defence. The skin cells begin to reproduce themselves dramatically so that the upper layers of skin coarsen and thicken to form a better barrier (leading to the 'leathery' skin commonly found in people from sunny climates). At the same time the cells are stimulated to produce melanin in order to protect the skin from burning. Although some melanin is present at the skin surface, it takes up to two days for extra quantities to be produced and distributed, by which time you can be already burned. Melanin's natural job at the skin surface is to filter out the sun's rays, so that a suntan is in effect a natural defence mechanism. It is when excess UVB rays pass through the skin and this natural protection mechanism can no longer cope, that you experience the agonies of sunburn.

SUCCESSFUL SUNTANNING

Whatever your skin type, there are several common-sense factors to bear in mind when sunbathing. Although it is tempting to spend all day every day in the sun when you only have a short holiday, do remember to proceed with caution especially at first, only exposing yourself to about 15 minutes sun on the first day, and then gradually increasing this time on subsequent days. The effects of the sun do not appear until several hours after exposure, so it is only too easy to become burned without being aware of it. Do beware, too, of a day which is windy or cloudy since both these weather conditions can lull you into a false sense of security, when in fact you could still get sunburned. It is also worth taking heed of that old saying about mad dogs and Englishmen going out in the midday sun. The sun is at its highest and its hottest between about noon and 2 pm, and especially if you are holidaying abroad, it is advisable to avoid the sun during this time.

Last but by no means least, do make sure to choose a really good suntanning preparation. This is one occasion when it is really not a good idea to use homemade products, since they do not contain the necessary sun filters.

Suntan products slow down the effect of the sun's rays, giving the skin time to activate melanin, so that you can tan without burning. Most products today screen out some of the UVB and the UVA rays.

Although you will find a bewildering array of suntan preparations on the shelves, most consist of oils (which may be vegetable or mineral), emulsified with water to moisturize the skin's outer layer and prevent it thickening, plus a chemical which acts as a sun filter. Some products are moisturizers only, so always read the label carefully. Chemicals are nearly always used as filtering agents, since naturally occurring ones are not only rare, but are also not effective on their own. The only exceptions are PABA (one of the B complex), umbelliferon (found in some plants) and salicylic acid (from willow bark), which can come from natural sources.

Some products sold in the health food shops incorporate a natural filter with a smaller amount of synthetics. If you are looking for a product that is as natural as possible, choose one based on plant oils such as sesame, jojoba, coconut, aloe vera, carnauba or cocoa butter. Mineral oils are said to be less effective in absorbing the sun's rays, and may even draw vitamins out of the tissues via the skin. Suntan products need to be blended with care since some of the tropical oils, such as bergamot and coconut, act as tan accelerators and can result in irregular colouration and may carry an increased cancer risk. Never use these oils neat, and steer clear of them if your skin is at all sensitive.

Today's suntan products invariably carry a number which indicates their sun protection factor (SPF). The higher the number, the greater the degree of protection afforded, but since there is no agreed standard, different brands can vary considerably. It is advisable to start with a high SPF number, and then move to a lower number as your skin becomes acclimatized.

A normal skin can use any of the suntanning preparations, whether it be oil, cream or lotion, although creams generally give better protection. If you have a dry skin it is best to use an oil which will help to moisturize the skin while protecting it. An oily skin, on the other hand, would do better with a light lotion. This is one time when a greasy skin comes into its own – it is likely to tan faster and become less dehydrated than other skin types. If you are prone to spots, you will also find that these improve after exposure to the sun.

Whatever suntanning product you choose, remember to apply it every couple of hours while you are sunbathing, and after swimming. Pay particular attention to your nose, shoulders, chest, the lower part of your stomach, and the tops of your legs. These are all danger areas which need extra applications of suncream to prevent burning. It is best to avoid wearing perfume, cologne or deodorant while you are sunbathing, since these can not only cause skin discolouration but also increase the absorption of sunlight by the skin.

Vitamin A is said to help prevent sunburn by building up the skin's own resistance more quickly than normal. Take extra vitamin A both before and during your holiday. While the level of vitamin A in the blood drops after intensive exposure to ultra violet rays, the production of vitamin D is encouraged. In sunnier climates than our own, the action of sunlight on the skin is often a major source of vitamin D, which is poorly distributed in foods. Sunbathing also depletes vitamin B levels, since these nutrients are involved in the production of melanin, so remember to pack your brewer's yeast tablets.

USING A SUNBED SAFELY

It can help to accustom your skin to the sun even before you set off on holiday, using the weaker rays of a sunbed. These are now available at many beauty salons and sports centres, but it is vital to adhere to the following safety precautions.

1. Always choose a sunbed which emits purely UVA rays. Some models offer a very fast tanning facility (sometimes in as little as ten minutes) but these are dangerous since they

have a high output of UVB rays.

2. A reputable salon or centre should offer you protective eye goggles (ultraviolet rays can cause severe eye strain, and even cataracts). They should also keep a medical record for you, checking before each session whether you suffered any adverse reaction the previous time; and they should warn you that certain drugs (such as the contraceptive pill and tranquillizers) increase the skin's sensitivity to light.

3. As with sunbathing on the beach, remove all cosmetics, perfumes or deodorants which may irritate the skin under the ultraviolet rays.

4. Always stick to the recommended exposure time for your type of skin—beds should be fitted with an automatic timer. Do not use the sunbed daily; limit your visits to three times a week until a tan is established, then once every one or two weeks.

5. If you develop a headache, itching, feel any discomfort or burning, or feel unwell in any other way either during or after use, stop at once.

6. As with proper sunbathing, you need to nourish your skin with a moisturizing oil or lotion after using a sunbed to counteract the drying effect of the ultraviolet light (see below).

REPLACING LOST MOISTURE
Because the sun has such a drying effect on the skin, it is essential to counteract this by applying lashings of moisturizer. Otherwise you may end up looking wrinkled and leathery – hardly the desired effect! You just cannot apply too much moisture while you are in the sun, even if your skin tends to be naturally greasy.

Make it a habit to moisturize your body all over every evening while on holiday, and add an oil to your bath water too. Each morning rub coconut oil all over yourself, and then wash it off in the shower or bath. Salt water aggravates the dryness, and should be washed off with fresh water as soon as possible, or at least every evening. When you return home, and your tan begins to fade along with your holiday memories, don't leave off the moisturizing treatment. It helps to preserve your tan by slowing up the natural shedding of the outer layers of skin, and discourages any peeling or flakiness.

If you do overdo the sunbathing and find yourself suffering the agonies of sunburn, an application of cider vinegar and water, of mashed cucumber, strong tea or milk helps to soothe the burn.

LOOKING AFTER YOUR HAIR
It is not just your skin which is likely to suffer on a sunny holiday. Salt water, sea breezes and sun also combine to play havoc with your hair. Always wash the salt water out at the end of the day, and wear a protective head-covering if the sun is very hot. This is particularly important if your hair is dyed or bleached, since the sun can often change the colour dramatically. Choose a rich cream shampoo, and follow this with a conditioner to put back the oils the sun has taken out. Even greasy hair will benefit from conditioning while you are on holiday. Although you need to rinse the salt water out of your hair, resist the temptation to shampoo it more often than usual.

PROTECTING YOUR EYES
Sunglasses are a good investment to protect your eyes from the harsh sunlight, especially if you find that the glare gives you a headache or causes you to screw up your eyes. This is particularly the case if you are near water, or in the snow, where you get a lot of reflection.

There are three types of glasses to choose from: tinted, polarized or photocromic/photomatic. Tinted glasses consist simply of tinted plastic or glass lenses which absorb some of the direct sunlight. Polarized glasses have a thin film of polarizing material sandwiched between two layers of plastic, and it is the chemical make up of the lens which serves to cut out the glare. Photocromic or photomatic glasses have light sensitive lenses. These contain crystals which react to the ultraviolet rays of the sun, so that the tint of the glasses changes as you move from sun to shade or vice versa.

IN COLDER CLIMATES
On a cold weather holiday, extra moisture and protection are again important, since the skin suffers from either extreme of temperature. Especially likely to suffer from the cold are dry or sensitive skins. Whatever your skin type, apply a rich moisturizer and a light foundation before venturing out into the cold. These will protect your face from the elements, and help prevent thread veins and an unsightly red nose. Apply a lip salve to stop your lips becoming sore and chapped, and use a rich hand cream and warm gloves to protect your hands. In the evenings after a day spent out in the cold, have a relaxing warm bath, followed by an all-over application of body lotion.

HOLIDAY BEAUTY CHECKLIST

Hot Weather Holiday

Suntanning preparation
Sunburn soother (just in case)
Moisturizer
Body Lotion
Bath oil
Headcovering
Brewer's yeast tablets
Vitamin A supplement
Rich cream shampoo
Hair conditioner

Cold Weather Holiday

Rich moisturizer
Light foundation cream
Lip salve
Body Lotion
Rich hand cream
Warm gloves

CHAPTER ELEVEN

HOME-MADE COSMETICS

Because cosmetics do not by law have to declare a list of ingredients, there is usually no way of telling just what has gone into a particular product. This means that some of the ingredients of the cosmetics you buy could, for all you know, be doing your skin more harm than good. This problem occurs particularly with those who are allergic to certain substances, and who have no way of knowing whether the offending ingredient is present in a given product.

One way to be sure of just what you are putting on your skin is to make your own cosmetics. It is an idea which will appeal to any do-it-yourself enthusiast or keen cook, but you don't need to be an expert in either of these fields to obtain enjoyment and success from making your own skin care products. As you will see from the suggestions later in this chapter, some of the ideas are so simple that a child could make them, and even the more complicated recipes are easily mastered if you follow the instructions through step by step.

Another plus point for home-made cosmetics is their cost. Those women for whom expensive cosmetics are out of reach have no excuse for neglecting their skin when so many household items can benefit the complexion. No expensive equipment is needed, and the few special ingredients you will have to buy are unlikely to break the bank, especially since they are used in very small quantities and so last a long time.

There is no point in making up gallons of a lotion or cream at one session. For one thing, unless you have tried a particular recipe before, you may find that it does not suit your particular skin. Since home-made cosmetics are made from fresh ingredients and without preservatives they also have a shorter life than bought products. If stored in airtight containers most cosmetics will keep for a month or two, by which time you have probably used them up anyway. However, a recipe containing any ingredients you would normally store in the refrigerator is best refrigerated. One of the advantages of making up small batches at a time is that you can afford to experiment with all sorts of different cosmetics – an experiment which would set you back a lot of money if you used shop products.

You should be able to obtain any of the special items mentioned in the following recipes from your chemist. However, in case of difficulty, John Bell and Croydon of Wigmore Street, London W1, should be able to help. Many recipes call for lanolin, which comes in two forms: either hydrous or anhydrous. The difference is that the anhydrous lanolin has no added water, while the hydrous has a high water content. The following recipes use anhydrous lanolin. The kind of oil you use in your cosmetics is governed by the type of skin you have. If your skin is greasy you are best advised to use mineral oil rather than vegetable oil, since this is less penetrating. For those with dry or normal skins, any kind of vegetable oil is suitable. Most of the recipes given here do not include any perfume, but if you want a more fragrant cosmetic, try adding a few drops of an essential oil such as lavender oil. These can be obtained from Baldwins, of 77 Walworth Road, London SE17.

COSMETICS FROM THE KITCHEN CUPBOARD

You may be surprised to learn that many of the ingredients you would normally have in your kitchen can also be used as natural beauty aids. To get yourself attuned to making your own cosmetics, start off by trying some of these simple ideas using household ingredients.

APPLES
Use as the basis for a dry skin face mask, or a hand lotion. Finely chop and mash an apple, then add half a teaspoonful of milk and a tablespoonful of honey.

BREWER'S YEAST POWDER
Used as an ingredient in a facial, this is good for the circulation. Don't use it more than once a week, and apply a thin coating of oil to the skin first. Because this mask can bring out impurities, avoid using it before going out anywhere special. Dissolve half a teaspoonful of yeast powder in a little water, and add a tablespoonful of honey, a tablespoonful of vegetable oil, and half a teaspoonful of cider vinegar. Mix well. If your skin is greasy, add a tablespoonful of yogurt, buttermilk or whipped egg white. For dry skins, add a tablespoonful of sour cream and one beaten egg yolk.

CIDER VINEGAR
Mixed with equal parts of water, this cleanses and tones the skin. If added to the final rinse water when washing the hair, it also helps eliminate dandruff and restores the hair's natural acid coating, which is usually removed by the shampoo. A cupful of cider vinegar in the bathwater is said to relieve aches and pains, while drinking a tablespoonful of cider vinegar in water three times a day before meals helps to strengthen finger nails.

CUCUMBER JUICE
This makes a good toner, or you can mash whole cucumber and use it as a toning face mask. Obtain cucumber juice by liquidizing and straining a chopped cucumber, or mash and sieve the cucumber. Cucumber does not keep well, so any product containing it should be stored under

refrigeration. Slices of cucumber placed over the eyes while you relax for 15 minutes help to refresh and soothe tired eyes.

EGG WHITE
Beaten and applied to a greasy skin as a face mask, egg white helps to refine large pores and tone the skin. To vary, add the juice of half a lemon.

EGG YOLK
Mixed with a tablespoonful of vegetable oil, this makes a good face mask for dry or sensitive skins. Make it more nourishing by adding a tablespoonful of honey. See page 89 for an egg yolk shampoo, or try the following: mix 1 egg with 1 to 2 tablespoonsful of herbal shampoo. Beat in a tablespoonful of gelatine for extra conditioning. Make a hair conditioner by beating together 3 egg yolks, and a few drops each of glycerine, cider vinegar and vegetable oil. Gently warm the mixture and apply it to your hair half an hour before shampooing.

GELATINE
This helps to set hair if added to final rinse water. Dissolve two tablespoonsful in two cups of boiling water before adding.

HONEY
This can be used on its own as a face mask for dry or normal skins. When combined with oatmeal it helps refine a greasy skin. To make a honey hair conditioner, beat one egg with a tablespoonful of honey and two teaspoonsful of vegetable oil. Massage into your hair, and leave on for half an hour before shampooing.

LEMON JUICE
Lemon juice mixed with an equal quantity of water or

rosewater tones and bleaches the skin. Add it to the final
rinse water when shampooing your hair, or comb or spray
on undiluted juice as a hair setting lotion.

MILK
A good skin cleanser when used in conjunction with a
proper cleanser. After cleansing the skin, wipe over with
cotton wool soaked in milk. Used in this way night and
morning it will keep the skin really clean, and help clear up
any blackheads or open pores.

OATMEAL
Fine oatmeal can be mixed with a little water and used as a
facial scrub to remove unwanted dead skin cells (see page
35). Mixed with honey, milk or water, oatmeal makes a
good cleansing and refining face mask. Oatmeal and/or
bran can be used as a dry shampoo, by rubbing well into
the hair and then brushing out thoroughly. For a cleansing,
soothing bath, tie a tablespoonful of bran or oatmeal in a
piece of muslin or cheesecloth and place in the bathwater.
Make a paste for washing with by combining a tablespoonful each of oatmeal, dried and ground orange peel, and
ground almonds. Add enough water to give a paste.

POTATOES
Grated raw and applied to the eye area, they help eliminate
puffiness and bags.

ROSEWATER AND WITCHHAZEL
These can be combined to make a simple toner. Use equal
quantities for a greasy skin, or 3/4 rosewater to 1/4
witchhazel for normal skin. If your skin is very dry, dilute
the toner with a little water.

SEA SALT
Sea salt dissolved in ice cold water or applied direct to the

wet skin refines open pores and helps to remove the surface layer of dead skin.

YOGURT
This makes a good cleanser for oily skins. It also helps to improve unmanageable hair if massaged well in for about three minutes after shampooing. Rinse out thoroughly.

SOME SIMPLE COSMETIC RECIPES

ALMOND HAND CREAM
½ oz. (12g) white wax
2 fl.oz. (50ml) rosewater
6 tablespoonsful almond oil
1 teaspoonful vegetable oil

Melt the wax and oils over hot water. Beat in the rosewater drop by drop, and continue beating until the mixture cools.

BUBBLE BATH
1 egg
1 teaspoonful gelatine
½ cupful herbal shampoo

Mix all the ingredients together with an electric whisk. Add to the bath water under the running tap.

CUCUMBER CLEANSER
3 teaspoonsful beeswax
5 teaspoonsful mineral oil
1 teaspoonful glycerine
4 tablespoonsful vegetable oil
4 tablespoonsful cucumber juice
Pinch of borax

Melt the oils and wax over hot water. Gently heat the rest of the ingredients together until the borax has dissolved. Add the borax mixture to the oils a drop at a time, stirring constantly. Beat until cool. Refrigerate.

CUCUMBER AND MINT TONING LOTION

½ cucumber
2 tablespoonsful witchhazel
4 tablespoonsful mint leaves
1 tablespoonful rosewater

Put all the ingredients into a liquidizer and blend until smooth. Store in a refrigerator.

HONEY MOISTURIZER

3 tablespoonsful lanolin
4 tablespoonsful warm water
½ tablespoonful honey

Melt the lanolin over hot water. Slowly add the honey and water, beating well. Remove from the heat and beat until cool. Do not refrigerate, or the cream may separate.

LEMON NOURISHING CREAM

2 eggs
1 teaspoonful lemon juice
2 beaten egg yolks
1 teaspoonful glycerine
2 teaspoonsful vegetable oil
2 tablespoonsful water

Blend the eggs, glycerine and lemon juice. Slowly add enough oil to give a thick cream. Add the egg yolks and water a little at a time, stirring constantly. Refrigerate.

LIME BODY LOTION

3 tablespoonsful rosewater
2 tablespoonsful lime juice
1 tablespoonful glycerine

Blend all the ingredients together. Use after a bath. This lotion is excellent for dry skin, and has the advantage of not being too oily.

MILK LOTION FOR ROUGH SKIN
½ pt. (275ml) milk
½ oz. (12g) bicarbonate of soda
½ oz. (12g) glycerine
½ oz. (12g) borax

Warm the milk and slowly add the other ingredients. Heat gently until the borax dissolves.

ROSE CLEANSING CREAM
2 teaspoonsful castile soap,
  grated
4 tablespoonsful lanolin
2 tablespoonsful oil
2 tablespoonsful rosewater
Pinch of borax (if needed)

Melt the soap with the oil and lanolin in a double boiler (a bowl over a pan of boiling water will do). Add the rosewater a little at a time, beating with a whisk. Remove from the heat and whisk until cool. If the mixture separates, whisk again, adding the borax. Pot and leave in the refrigerator to set.

SUMMER TONER WITH RASPBERRIES
2 cupsful raspberries
1 teaspoonful honey
1 cupful rose petals
2 pt. (1¼litre) cider vinegar

Steep the raspberries and rose petals in the cider vinegar and honey for a month. Strain and add an equal quantity of water.

VITAMIN E EYE CREAM

1 tablespoonful lanolin
2 teaspoonsful cold water
1½ tablespoonsful almond oil
1 vitamin E capsule

Melt the lanolin and oil over hot water. Remove from the heat and add the water and the contents of the vitamin E capsule. Beat well with an electric mixer or wooden spoon. This gives quite a runny cream.

CHAPTER TWELVE

AN INTRODUCTION TO THE BEAUTY WORLD

Trends in beauty and cosmetics are continually changing, but apart from the occasional appearance of a new and wonderful beauty aid, the basic principles and ingredients remain the same. This chapter serves as an introduction to some of the ingredients you are likely to find, to some of the special terms used, and to some of the beauty treatments currently on offer.

HOW PRODUCTS ARE MADE

Emulsion: a combination of two liquids that do not normally dissolve in each other, but are blended with the aid of an emulsifier. These are either oil in water (fine particles of water dispersed in fat or oil) or water in oil. Most creams and lotions are emulsions, but lotions have a higher water content than creams.

Hypoallergenic: less likely to cause a reaction but cannot guarantee no reaction. Such products are usually unscented, with formulae that are as simple as possible, and exclude common sensitizers such as lanolin (see below).

Medicated: a specific action beyond the normal cleansing, toning or deodorizing. For instance, additives like benzoyl peroxide or salicylic acid increase grease-removing properties of some soaps, while zinc pyrithione and selenium sulphide may be used in antiperspirants. The medicated products are harsher and more likely to cause sensitivity or allergy.

Preservatives: any product which is going to last a reasonable length of time will contain some preservatives.

These are in the form of antioxidants (to prevent contamination from exposure to air); anti-bacterial compounds (to prevent or discourage the growth of bacteria or moulds); stabilizers with anti-bacterial properties (to combine the qualities of the first two categories, thereby making them the best preservatives).

Soapless shampoos and cleansing products: these have not been saponified, i.e. made into soap by mixing natural animal or vegetable oils with an alkali such as potassium. Instead they combine lanolin, oils, colouring, perfume and protein.

Superfatted soaps: unsaponified fat is left in the soap during processing, or lanolin, glycerine, beeswax or mineral oils are added to a soap base. These rich soaps are designed for dry or mature skins, but are less effective as cleansers because of the inclusion of non-cleansing ingredients.

Unscented products: unless a product actually states that it has no perfume added it will probably contain a scent or group of scents. These are usually used in a very low concentration (e.g. 0.5 per cent), but even so perfumes are one of the most common causes of adverse reaction.

Vanishing cream: an oil-in-water emulsion which penetrates the skin without leaving an oily film on the surface.

NATURAL INGREDIENTS

Almonds: high in polyunsaturates. Almond oil has a particular affinity with the skin and helps protect its acid/alkaline balance.

Aloe Vera: a gel-like juice from a spiky cactus-type plant, a member of the lily family, a succulent perennial growing wild in tropical and sub tropical climates. The gel has been used over several thousand years for its healing properties, especially in the treatment of wounds, burns and skin irritations. Research programmes conducted in both America and Russia substantiate these claims. It also acts as an efficient moisturizer, with the ability to penetrate deeply into the dermal layers of the skin.

Apricot: a member of the almond family (see above), and high in vitamin A. The oil, which is obtained from the kernel of the fruit, is rich in trace enzymes, minerals and vitamin A. Helps to soften the skin and preserve natural moisture content.

Avocado: especially good for dry skin because it is rich and moisturizing. It contains beta carotene (a form of vitamin A), vitamins D and E, all of which are good for the skin.

Beeswax: traditionally used as a base for other cosmetic ingredients. Creams containing it tend to be rich and heavy, and so especially suited to dry or mature skins.

Calendula: the official name for the marigold, this has been used for centuries to assist in healing, especially of skin infections such as acne. A concentrated tincture or oil is used, both of which are obtained from the flower.

Chamomile: a herb which is soothing and anti-inflammatory, thus especially helpful in treating swelling or sores. A natural bleaching agent, so often used in products for fair hair (see page 90).

Cocoa butter: this was once a very popular cosmetic ingredient, but is less frequently used now. It is a solidified oil from the roasted cocoa bean, and is thick and heavy in texture. It is especially good in suntan preparations since it helps screen the skin from the burning rays of the sun.

Comfrey: known as a medicinal herb since Roman times, and until the 17th century used mainly for healing bones (which earned it the nickname of 'knitbone'). Both the root and leaves are used in the preparation of cosmetics, comfrey being particularly valued as a healer, a skin softener and a moisturizer.

Collagen: a relatively new arrival on the cosmetic market, this is a form of protein obtained from animals (e.g. from placenta and plasma). It is constructed of fibres, and gives firmness and resilience to the skin. Its creamy texture makes it useful as an emollient (i.e. softener), to prevent moisture loss and to plump out wrinkles.

Elastin: this is similar to collagen in that it is also an animal protein structure and the chief ingredient of the elastic tissue in the skin. It works well with wrinkles, giving the skin more elasticity.

Essential oils: unadulterated oils extracted from plants in minute quantities. Ideal for adding perfume to natural cosmetics, but they are very expensive, not surprising when you consider that a kilo of rose petals, and a complicated distillation process, are necessary to produce one small bottle of rose oil. Cheaper versions are available with a small amount of an essential oil diluted in almond oil. The essential oils are the ones used by aromatherapists to cure a wide range of health and beauty problems. They are massaged into the affected area or inhaled, where they are believed to take a direct route to the brain and the central nervous system. Therapists claim that just the fragrance can calm the nerves and soothe aches and pains, while the oil can penetrate the skin and enter the bloodstream in order to cure minor ailments. The oils certainly have antiseptic properties.

Henna: (see page 91) comes from the lawsonia plant which grows in Africa and Asia. The plant is picked, dried in the sun and then crushed into a powder.

Jojoba: one of the latest wonders of the beauty world, this is said to surpass any other animal or vegetable oil for use on the skin, and it has the added advantage of being an ideal substitute for sperm whale oil which is now banned. The oil is extracted from the bean of a small shrub which grows in desert areas, where the local people have used the oil for hundreds of years both for the hair and the skin. The plant itself is amazing, in that it grows in the most extreme hot arid conditions, it takes 10 years to reach maturity, and then goes on to produce about 10 lbs of nuts every year for up to 100 years. This pure, golden oil, which differs dramatically from other known plant oils, is non toxic, does not go rancid, needs no chemical refining and remains chemically unchanged for years. Jojoba is gentle and non-irritant and makes an excellent moisturizer, being easily absorbed by the skin. It also helps improve hair and scalp condition. Quite apart from its uses in the cosmetic field, the oil is also used for coating pills, as a soothing agent in disinfectants, as a lubricant in open heart surgery and in manufacturing industries of many kinds. In fact, jojoba was voted one of the top ten investments of the 1980s by the *Wall Street Digest*, and research is currently being conducted in both America and Japan on other uses for it. Jojoba was tested using the LD50 method of testing (see page 10) in America in 1979.

Keratin: a protein compound which also forms the main ingredient of our nails and hair. A simple laboratory process extracts it from animal or human hair, and it is included in hair care products for its apparent ability to strengthen and build.

Lanolin: a natural oil which is obtained from sheep's wool. It is an emollient (i.e. softener), and it acts as an emulsifier and is often used as the base for creams and lotions. Especially good for dry skins.

Rosemary: used for centuries for its pungent essential oil. It has refreshing and astringent properties, and is particularly recommended for improving hair strength and growth.

Sage: The plant's chief active ingredients are essential oils and tannins which have antiseptic and astringent properties and stimulate the circulation. Enlivens the skin and scalp, has cleansing and deodorising abilities, and helps reduce open pores.

Vitamin E: a natural antioxidant, which means it can help protect cells from damage and breakdown. Assists cell respiration and the formation of new cells, and helps protect the oils already present in the cells. Used principally to help keep the skin looking young and healthy, and also to assist in healing.

Witchhazel: a traditional remedy dating back hundreds of years, and obtained from the bark of an American tree. Renowned for its astringent and anti-inflammatory properties.

PERFUMES
It is virtually impossible to tell what has gone into a particular perfume, because it could contain as many as 50 different ingredients. It will undoubtedly have gone through a complicated process of selecting and blending to obtain the desired scent – a process which can take years, because you often need a whole mixture just to obtain one particular note of a perfume; for instance, a pure rose scent is never just rose essence.

Basically a perfume is a mixture of neat perfume oil, water and pure alcohol. Unless a perfumier states that he concentrates on natural ingredients (usually flower fragrances), it is difficult to tell where his perfume extracts come from. Even natural perfume oils may have had other natural or man-made oils added to give them the consistency which is otherwise only found in synthetic oils.

Your best chances of finding a natural perfume are to go

for one of the expensive well known French producers, or for one of the smaller houses specializing in natural flower scents, but even then there are no guarantees that a perfume is free from synthetics, although such companies do aim for a greater proportion of natural ingredients.

The perfume industry used to rely on a lot of animal ingredients, but this is less common today, mainly because of the prohibitive cost. For instance, common animal fixatives are musk (from a Himalayan deer), ambergris (from sperm whales) and civet (from the glands of civet cats kept in small cages). If a reasonably priced perfume calls itself musk it is extremely unlikely to contain the real thing, but instead will be produced synthetically.

All perfumes contain some alcohol, with most in the concentrated scents, and less in the lighter perfumes which have a higher proportion of water (and so last less long). If you are sensitive to alcohol on your skin, an alternative is an oil based perfume such as an essential oil (where a pure plant oil is diluted in vegetable oil). A cheap perfume oil, on the other hand, will undoubtedly be based on mineral oil.

Before buying any perfume always test it on your skin first, since perfumes react differently on various people. Natural perfumes tend to last less well than the cheap synthetic ones. Wear your perfume at the pulse points where the body temperature is slightly warmer, encouraging evaporation and allowing the full scent to develop. These are around the hairline, behind the ears, the nape of the neck, under the breasts, in the crook of the arm and inside the wrists.

BEAUTY TREATMENTS
The following treatments are usually on offer at a beauty salon, but if you want to find one which makes use of natural beauty products your best bet is to opt for one of the smaller, independent salons. It is always advisable to

pay a visit to a salon before you make an appointment, to enquire about what products and equipment they use, and if you are particularly concerned about whether their products are natural or not, it is as well to ask to see an ingredients list, because their interpretation of natural may be very different from yours.

Cleansing: a very thorough, deep cleansing which leaves the skin feeling fresher and softer, and is sure to remove all accumulated grime and dead skin cells.

Electrical treatments: these are fairly extreme, and so are only used where essential and must be given with great care. Of help to dry and mature skins since the skin can be made temporarily more absorbent, so that helpful substances can be absorbed at a deeper level than normal. Also useful for removing excess sebum from oily skins.

Face mask: various different forms are used, but look for one that is soft and gentle, perhaps including herbs, fruits or yogurt.

Facial massage: guaranteed to make you feel good if performed by an experienced masseuse. Relieves muscular tensions.

Laser: A gentle beam with a comparatively low frequency is used to stimulate skin cells, thereby ironing out wrinkles and plumping out ageing skin. Also used in the treatment of problems like cellulite, acne scars, eczema and psoriasis.

Skin peeling: removes the surface layer of dead skin cells which makes the skin look dull. The most natural method is the biological, in which a product with a granular texture is used (like the method described on page 35).

Steaming: a machine directs steam at the face from a short distance. This oxygenates the skin cells, acting as a cleanser, speeding up skin renewal and increasing circulation of blood to the skin.

During treatment the operator holds what looks like a fat metal pencil on to the point requiring treatment (it in fact works on the main trigger points as does acupuncture). Treatment lasts about 20 minutes, and the most you should feel is a slight tingling. The laser beam penetrates no more than 2mm beneath the skin's surface, but this is enough to stimulate the cells to work harder and to rejuvenate skin tissue faster than normal. There are four safety classifications for lasers: class 1 which is totally safe (for instance those used to read bar codes in supermarkets); class 2 which can be damaging although the body's defence system can usually cope; class 3, a more concentrated beam which is not safe to look at directly; class 4 which is for heavy medical use only. Beauticians will be using those in any of the first three classifications, and because of the potential risks it is essential to check that the treatment is given by fully trained personnel.

INDEX